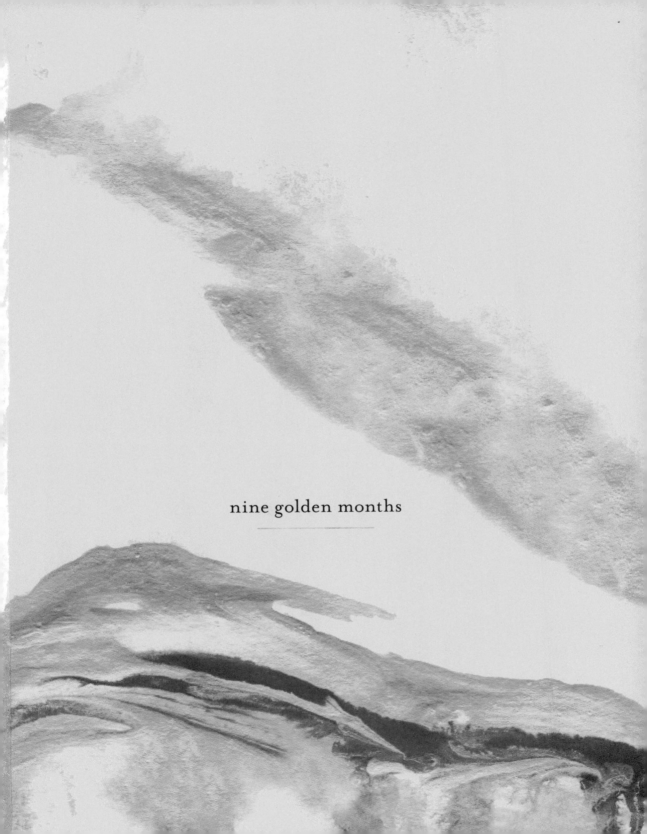

nine golden months

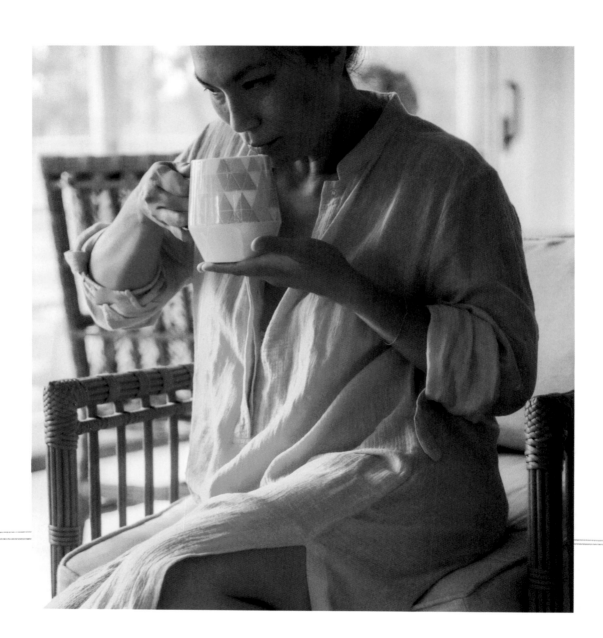

nine golden months

The Essential Art of
Nurturing the Mother-to-Be

HENG OU

AMELY GREEVEN AND MARISA BELGER

ABRAMS IMAGE, NEW YORK

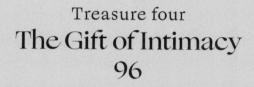

INTRODUCTION

Congratulations! You are pregnant, creating a baby and growing a new life. Your entire being is at its creative peak, and you are expanding in so many ways. Physically, it's quite awe inspiring, as your womb stretches from mere inches to watermelon size. Psychically, it's equally so. Your heart may feel like it is exploding in every direction— feeling more love and hope than you ever thought possible in some moments, more doubt and worry in others. Your mind may be blown by the scope of the responsibility you are taking on, and your very sense of who you are may be starting to shift, as the woman you have known for decades shakes free of her old foundations to allow a new you to emerge: Mother. (Or as the case may be, Mother Again.)

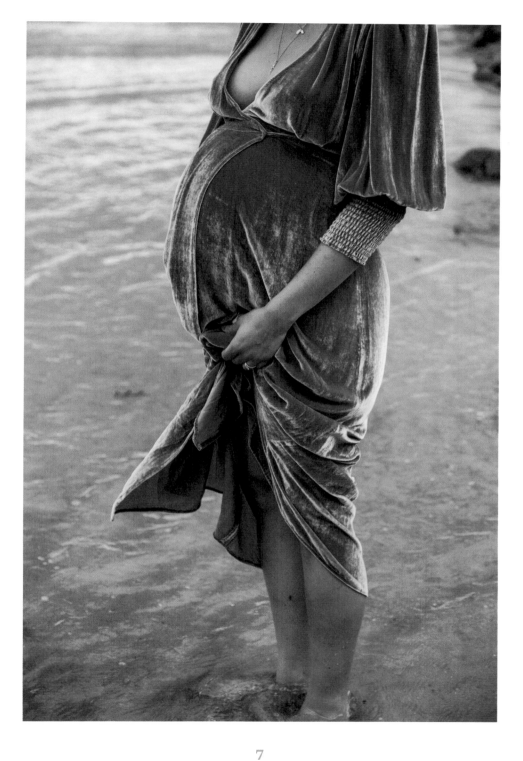

Being pregnant is a phenomenon unlike any other. When else in your life will you experience three-quarters of a year of such constant construction, the around-the-clock building project that is making a baby—and destruction, as old ways of being (in the world, in your body, in your relationship) fall away to reveal the next chapter of you? Imagine reading an epic tale in which the protagonist is pushed to the very edges of her physical and mental capacity and thrust into the depths of devotion and surrender before discovering a bond unlike any other. That person is you, playing the starring role in the most monumental story of creation and evolution that exists—it is epic! The changes that you are experiencing in your body, and in your mind and emotions as well, are breathtaking.

But chances are that by and large, the rest of the world is not changing much for you. Sure, at the peak of pregnancy—with your gloriously rounded belly telegraphing "Baby on board"—strangers may beam smiles or offer their seats on the bus. As your due date approaches, the well wishes pick up, and gifts and hand-me-downs may arrive from family and friends. And ads for must-have baby items or next-level nursing bras might mysteriously pop up in your social media feeds. But, curiously, for such a massive undertaking—one human creating an entirely new life-form and birthing that being into the world—you might be discovering that society at large emanates a strange sense of nonchalance. Pregnancy for the most part elicits a "Move along, nothing to see here" kind of attitude in our culture. Sure, we will get out the streamers when baby actually arrives, and yes, we will tell you how proud we are of what you have just done when you send the birth announcement out. But until the evidence is front and center (all adorable teeny fingers and piercing cries), life's pretty much as normal. Why shouldn't it be? After all, women can do it all!

But should we? In many cultures and in many times, and in many families and maternal lineages, the nine and a half months of pregnancy are recognized as anything but a normal time. They are an extraordinary time! And they deserve an extraordinary level of recognition and care. Not just for the baby within, but—very significantly—for the one doing the heavy lifting, transforming, and growing: mom herself.

If you are setting out, hopeful and hustling busily, on your pregnancy path today, you might be too occupied to consider that there is more to the experience. Before you conceived, your existence may have been anchored in place by daily to do's and goals to be met. Now, pregnancy's three trimesters of checkups, tests, classes, and home improvement projects can easily add to the load. If you let it, this essential period of your life can be reduced to a sequence of milestones asking to be met, carrying you along toward the ultimate project deadline: giving birth. And while it's true that if you stay on track with the tasks, you'll eventually come to an end point—meeting your baby for the first time—it's a shame to let this linear approach be all that you know. Pregnancy is all of that, but it is also so much more.

The thirty-eight-ish weeks of carrying a baby to term is a season of life that contains tremendous, even life-transforming, opportunities. Pregnancy and its zenith—the hours or days of labor and birth—will ask you to tap more strength than you ever knew you had as you face hard decisions, make risk assessments, and navigate monumental physical output. And you may find yourself doing all of this while allowing a vulnerability you may barely have permitted before. It deepens your sensitivity to everything around you, physically and emotionally, and enhances your intuition in almost mind-bending ways. And as many a teary-eyed mama can attest, gestating a child can bring long-stored feelings up to the surface, allowing tensions and fears to fully unravel and release, maybe for the very first time. Pregnancy can be a time of tremendous development for your baby, and great healing for you as well.

And that's not even touching on how pregnancy can be a spiritual initiation of sorts, introducing you to the creative power of the universe that lives inside your womb, and forever altering your sense of what your badass woman-self can do! Society never sees the superhero under their ordinary garb, and it's the same with you, clad in your maternity jeans. Most are oblivious to the astonishing force that you are, building a human being from two tiny cells, gearing up to bring another citizen into the world, permanently changing the shape of your family and yourself—all while juggling the demands of your job or meeting every need of your older kids. So while you may win some admiring comments about your slowly changing silhouette, you likely won't be congratulated for being born into the fierce and tender, generous and constant, and—from the highest perspective—powerfully enlightening experience of motherhood. Let's just say, pregnancy's labyrinth—as one of the wise women featured in this book describes it—is profound, paradoxical, and one of the most significant rites of passage in your life.

So why are we not shouting this part from the rooftops, or at least conveying it equally as enthusiastically as we do the news on prenatal vitamins and the

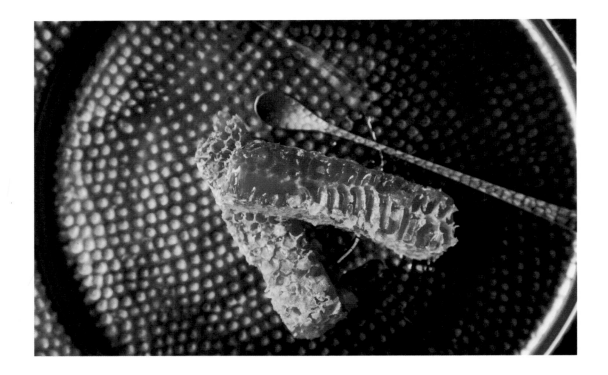

risks of smoking and drinking, or the latest on how to handle varicose veins and stretch marks?

The answer may partly lie in the way pregnancy and birth have become more of a prognosis, and a business, than a transformative rite. Starting in the twentieth century, the mechanistic model of care for pregnant women took hold. Under this model, largely male dominated at first, medical authorities began to "treat" pregnancy and delivery like many other medical conditions, with diagnoses, interventions, and standardized, clinic-based care. Swift and efficient, and financially lucrative, this linear model began eclipsing a more holistic approach, in which midwives and other elders in the community helped the natural cycles of prenatal, labor and delivery, and postpartum care run smoothly and a little differently for each mother. And while there's much to honor about this evolution—it has brought a level of safety to many mothers who might otherwise have been at risk, and offered dedicated medical care to families in need—it has also reframed things. The push toward ever more profitable medical treatments has forced the focus of care to get smaller and smaller, no longer encompassing the whole of the pregnant person's experience, and now overwhelmingly zeroed in on the baby itself. And the quiet side effect is that sometimes *you* can feel oddly left out of the process.

If you are pregnant as you read this, you may have experienced some of this linear reality already. As you slide into your scheduled appointment—a straight-backed chair catching you in the clinic's waiting room—desk-staff quickly offer clipboards and a pen. Insurance cards and paperwork change hands in a flurry. Well-trained nurses track your vitals and chart your physical stats. Bright lights keep your alertness high, and machines you're not quite familiar with are placed on or near your body, helping your doctor or physician's assistant make assessments about the progress in there—Baby's looking good; keep doing what you're doing. Dietary handouts are stapled and offered. The next appointment is put on the calendar and *whoosh*, you're on your way! Typically, it's been only a brief interruption to your daily programming.

Yet as you are moved through this system, treading its safe but slightly sterile terrain, a small voice inside may be making itself heard: What about me?

You see, the care that a mother-to-be needs during this time exceeds what the average clinical checkup can deliver. Being supported while carrying a baby is not only about eating off a prescribed list, cutting out alcohol, or editing harsh chemicals from her cleaning supplies—though these things matter. It's so much richer, more layered and textured than this. And it starts by turning inward.

When you allow yourself to sink into the care that expecting mothers need and deserve, you enter a realm beyond the measurable and quantifiable. Below that busy surface is a different kind of space, one where the mother feels safe, supported, and relaxed enough for her stress levels to stay low and for the distractions to subside, and where she can hear her inner knowing enough to trust it. A space where she can press pause on hyperproductivity and performing consistently "on the mark," and is permitted to feel differently from one day to the next. Where she naps when she needs to and turns off the world when she can—allowing, rather than resisting, her hormones' shifting rhythms of activity and rest. And where she has someone—or a few someones—who hold a mirror to the tremendous capacity that her body has, and who fully see her during all that pregnancy entails, from the triumphant top-of-the-world occasions to the moments of sleep-wrecking discomfort or doubt.

When a woman is allowed to be in this space, pregnancy becomes so much more than just a means to a (glorious) end—having a child. The pregnancy itself, including whatever kind of birth that she and her baby experience, becomes tremendously meaningful; a season of growing into her deserving power, and maturing into wisdom that forever changes how she embarks on mothering.

This is more important than ever today. At the time of writing, a perfect storm of factors—a global health and economic crisis, workplace closures, and in some places, local lockdowns too—are making a time of more isolation, not less, of more noise and more anxiety, not less. It has caught many women, their partners, and the pregnancy and birth workers who support them quite off guard. (Because how, really, could anyone prepare for this?) Nobody should be navigating the life-changing transition into parenthood deprived of touch or the simple gift of sitting with a dear friend as you sip hot bowls of soup. We need to place our newborns in the arms of trusted friends and family so we can take a shower or a nap. We need in-person solidarity and support. But that is exactly what is missing. Added to this, for many mothers of color in the US, pregnancy brings with it heightened—or even acute—anxiety about bringing a child into the world. This is a kind of fear that many other parents will simply never understand. All of this has been making the initiatory path that pregnant women walk into a full-on heroine's journey, one that demands they dig extra deep.

These circumstances may be extreme, but a silver lining gleams brightly. These intense times are forcing us to confront just how little, as a society, we lavish deep and meaningful care on women as we go through the most radically demanding and vulnerable transition of our lives. It's a fundamental misalignment, and it is at odds with what, from a holistic worldview, is practically a natural law: An expecting mother should never have to feel depleted, alone, or in any way adrift.

Which is where this book comes in. *Nine Golden Months* is a fluid, inclusive offering that weaves together many cords and threads, with food, wisdom, memories, and rituals for the pregnant person, circling around, intersecting and overlapping, and dancing with each other in their own nonlinear way. It came into being in a circuitous manner too, by being the third in a series of books devoted to what I see as a lost but essential art: mothering the mother during the months and years around conceiving and birthing a child. My first book in this series—the oldest sister in this family, so to speak—is *The First Forty Days: The Essential Art of Nourishing the New Mother*. On its release in 2016, *The First Forty Days* made the case for reclaiming the kind of dedicated, mother-centric postpartum care I had experienced at the hands of the Chinese medicine healers in my family, but that had been sadly forgotten in the rush of contemporary life. It offered a hybrid approach, rooted in time-honored methods, yet refreshed and reinvented to meet the way women live today. And it established a principle that defines how I live and work today: The mother is the central axis of the family. When she tips into depletion and lack—of nourishment, of rest, and of feeling seen and heard—the whole family can start to tip off its center.

The First Forty Days will always be my cherished firstborn—book-wise, that is! The *F40D* (to use its nickname) launched a movement to reclaim a vital missing piece of maternal care and lifted and elevated our collective expectations of what mothers deserve to receive. Its younger sister, *Awakening Fertility: The Essential Art of Preparing for Pregnancy*, came next, jumping back a little in the process—or forward to the next baby, as the case may be. It began a similar conversation about the crucially important, but often overlooked, preconception period, and offered a new way for women to feel held and supported as they prepared physically, mentally, and spiritually to conceive a child. These two books, filled with recipes that I developed in the kitchens of MotherBees, my maternal nourishment company, have helped new and growing families enjoy a level of resiliency and well-being they tell me they otherwise would not have had. And they have brought me and my dear friends and partners on the series—the wonderful writers Amely Greeven and Marisa Belger, and talented photographer Jenny McNulty—a sense of connectedness to women around the world that inspires, moves, and encourages us to keep creating, every single day.

For a spell, I felt these two literary daughters had made me complete. Though there was undeniably something missing in between conception and postpartum—quite a major missing link, in fact!—the subjects of pregnancy and childbirth seemed exceedingly well covered. Did the world need another pregnancy book, I wondered? Yet it's funny how siblings can come in. Sometimes they have their plan to arrive—their soul's contract, as some call it—no matter what you, the parent, logically think should occur. In this case, the profound conversations we were having with the pregnant and birthing women we knew—including Jenny, who'd just birthed her gorgeous daughter Marilla—helped Marisa, Amely, and me sense a third book wanting to be born. Despite the volumes of information already covering everything to expect about pregnancy from its first day until its last, a certain kind of wisdom about caring deeply for oneself along the way is still being lost.

That wisdom is what this book aims to capture. *Nine Golden Months* does not try to tell you which choices to make—and there are many of them, from early-day decisions around care providers and diagnostic tests to later-in-the-game ones about birth plans and placenta encapsulation (not to mention newborn diapers and tiny little sleep sacks!). Rather, it empowers you to discover and trust your own inner knowing of the choices you want to make to help create your ideal pregnancy and birthing experience, and it also holds you in a circle of intentional care, so that you can connect to the deeper story of your pregnancy that lies below the surface. It puts the onus not so much on preparing your environment for baby, but on doing the inner work of preparing to become the next version of yourself. Consider this book the companion to the existing array of excellent advice you may already be reading. It exists to feed you in all the ways that you deserve to be fed as you ride the highs and lows of pregnancy and fortify yourself for the momentous act of giving birth. Its purpose is to strengthen, embolden, and soothe you from the inside out; to help you avoid the dreaded state of maternal depletion at all costs; and to offer what may be the most important part of pregnancy care that can get lost in all the noise—the part about how *you* are doing and feeling as you are transforming into a mother!

In the pages that follow, you'll be invited to consider this question: What does it look like to truly mother myself while pregnant? For me this starts, as it does at any time on the mothering path, rather simply: with the food in your bowl, on your plate, and in your mug. Food takes on a whole new set of meanings when you are expecting—it is sometimes your best friend, other times your worst enemy. You crave it madly in some moments, and despair of how you'll ever face it again in others. Which means it helps if your relationship to what you eat is fluid, allowing, and compassionate (rather than restricting, fixed, or punishing). In this book, eating for pregnancy and birth is not presented as a clinical or nutritional lesson. Rather, I want to help ensure that the meals you make for yourself and your family become a reliable way to respond to your body's changing needs; to maintain a state of balance physically, mentally, and emotionally; and to fill your reserves as your body performs its most creative act. Inspired by the many meals my MotherBees kitchen has served to new mothers and mothers-to-be in California, I have crafted more than fifty nourishing and soothing recipes that are extremely simple and easy to execute, because you are already doing so very much. You will find my best tricks for tending discomforts too (like bouts of nausea and heartburn). And you'll find that the meals and drinks have been lovingly created to enchant your senses—taking you out of the mundane for a minute and even, I hope, into the magical. I believe cooking and eating are opportunities to take pause, anchor into the present moment, and connect deeply inside. My wish is that these recipes help you enjoy the ritual of eating in this unpredictable time. The recipes also help other people take care of you. They are easy for anyone to follow—and I implore you to ask people who love you to do exactly that. As a pregnant woman, you deserve to be lovingly, consistently, deliciously fed!

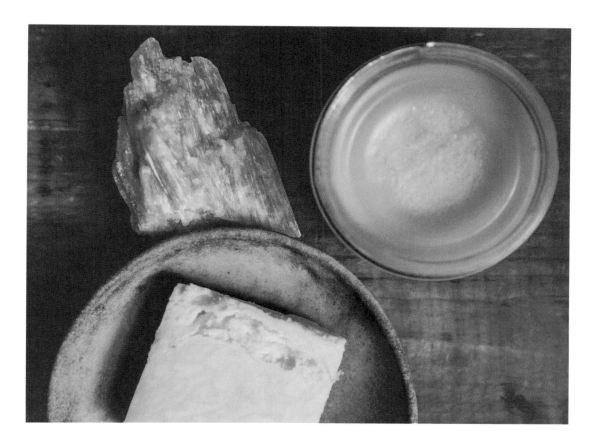

Much like *The First Forty Days* and *Awakening Fertility*, the recipes exist in a broader universe of care that mimics how it might feel to have the village—or at least a small circle—of wise, compassionate elders around you, people who have traversed this terrain many times before you. These are our book's "wise ones"— experienced birth workers, healers, and parents (and sometimes all three in one) who share with you what they share with those under their care, and in so doing, pass the flame of encouragement and empowerment around all things pregnancy and birth from one expecting person to the next. In a world full of advice about what you should do during this period of your life, the sections of the book before the recipes aim to support you in how to be: to cultivate a calm and confident inner state that buoys you through the parts of pregnancy that feel unpredictable. Fear not! These chapters will not add more tasks to your list; they give you reflections, inspirations, and small and simple practices to try when you have time. It's worth doing so. The insights will help you remember that, even when you're faced with another cold waiting room or you're pushing through another bout of heartburn, it is possible to reconnect to the wonder of what is occurring and to know, from your very core, that you are far from alone. So many women have passed through these same thresholds before you, and so many will after you.

Note: We care deeply about the experience of all people and write this book from a place of true inclusivity. In the text you will find the words "woman," "she/her," and "mother," as well as the term "pregnant people." We understand that becoming a parent is not limited by the confines of gender and write with open hearts, encircling and supporting the experiences of all pregnant and birthing people.

Don't get me wrong; I understand that the pregnancy experience is not all sunshine and rainbows. Not every woman floats through the (around) forty weeks of it happy and glowing. And even the most glowing among us will have hard days. Pregnancy can feel like a series of contradictory moments, and it can include bumps, hurdles, and downright challenges. You might be entering into childbearing feeling rested and ready as can be, or landing in it stunned by what's occurring—perhaps that it is happening at all. You might feel ablaze with feminine superpowers today and totally at odds with your radically morphing physique tomorrow. You might spend days, weeks, or even, sometimes, months in significant discomfort—though rest assured, the wise ones in this book have tremendous success in helping mothers avoid extreme depletion and distress when their balanced approach is followed. Becoming a mother inevitably includes profound challenge, and it can sometimes threaten to break your heart. One moment (such as birthing your baby) your resilience is tested to the limit; the next—like when you hold your newborn infant to your heart—your faith and self-belief skyrocket. This is the unacknowledged heart of the pregnancy and birth experience: You can be well researched, prepared, and grounded, but you can never fully control how events turn out. All you can do is take complete charge of your inner state of being, which is the very thing that gets you through it best.

There's no point dancing around it. Being pregnant means passing through the most heightened forms of human experiences—of love and hope, as well as doubt, fear, and even, sometimes, grief and loss. It holds in it everything, sometimes all at once, and it often can turn the volume up on all these states past comfortable levels—though many women go into pregnancy unaware of this possibility because nobody around them has brought it up. As we said in *F4OD*, the only way out is through. And when you can practice staying present through all of the sensations and feelings, grounded in a well-nourished, balanced body, feeling safe and supported and open to receiving help from others, then you do make it through and discover that even the hardest parts bring meaning to your story. Simply by balancing the busy preparation and appointments with a little bit of consistent inner attention, pregnancy can become a sacred experience.

It is considered an honor in many cultures to tend to a pregnant woman; it is thought that her every word, her every action is sacred. May you feel us honoring you, dear mother—for if you are pregnant, you are already a mother—as you immerse in the pages to come, or as you sink your hands into bowls of red jujubes to add to replenishing teas or inhale freshly sliced ginger to add to a hot pan. May you feel us holding a vision for your months of expectation: that you live deeply in this precious, fleeting experience; claim your primal birthing power; and stand in the fullness of your feminine force by the time this extraordinary voyage ends. You deserve nothing less than to start your mothering from this place! All we ask is that with this flame ignited, you pass the flame—perhaps via this book and its sisters!—forward to the next woman, so she can pass it forward to the next.

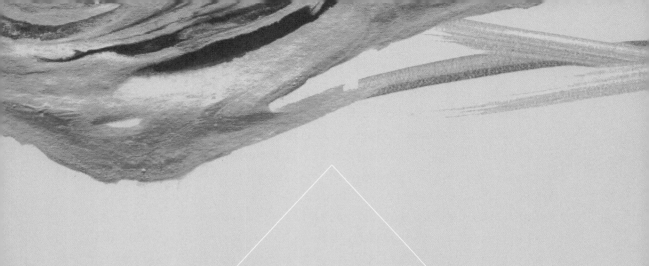

Reclaiming Our Right to Be Held

When I first became pregnant, almost twenty years ago now, I did not know I could create my own pregnancy experience or write its story. I was relatively young—in my late twenties—and living temporarily in the United Kingdom, and I launched into it the way most others around me did: at the local clinic, with well-intentioned yet time-pressed professionals taking my vitals, measuring how far along I was, and giving me stapled lists of what to do and not. I was very grateful this care was free, yet as a first-generation Taiwanese immigrant to the United States who'd been raised around traditional Chinese medicine healers, it was a bit of an odd fit.

The influence of my acupuncturist and herbalist aunties and uncle, as well as my maternal grandmother, Tu-Quyen—herself the granddaughter-in-law of a renowned doctor of Chinese medicine, Dr. Huang, in Vietnam—had made listening inward second nature. I'd become used to sinking into myself to note fluctuations in my body's temperature, shifts in my emotional state, or changes in my mindset, and then making adjustments to food, sleep, and lifestyle to smooth out any imbalances. Although they had not overtly stated it—my aunties are highly pragmatic and my grandmother was soft-spoken and restrained—I'd absorbed from them the understanding that health was an art. You did it with a kind of intuitive and often cyclical flow. It didn't look the same from person to person and it shape-shifted a bit from day to day.

Yet here I was on the cusp of one of the biggest "health events" of my life, and what I was experiencing didn't feel much like an art at all! Under bright fluorescent lights, my care providers efficiently moved me along the track: first appointment, second, third; tests scheduled, data gathered. The pregnancy books in the waiting room were full of expert opinion on what to expect and what to do about it, step by step. I'd never been one to follow structured systems. Frankly, as the Chinese kid thrown in to navigate midwestern elementary schools, or even later as an artistic teen who didn't fit the high school norm, I'd never even really understood systems. Setting out across the nine-month-long pregnancy landscape with the map fully written by others—*Everyone does it this way, Heng, just keep your head down and make it to the finish line*—felt oddly unsettling to me.

Plus, I had a secret I couldn't quite voice in those rushed prenatal visits. I was obsessed with pregnancy and birth! Long before actually becoming pregnant, I'd flip through hippie birth books and revel in the illustrations of babies in utero. I'd thrill to the details of week-by-week changes that mama and babe made together. A human, making their great masterpiece, in beautiful, cyclical phases! This was sheer magic in my mind. But magic and masterpieces, along with intuition and nature, didn't seem to have a place in the pregnancy journey I was about to take. It was two decades ago—the "divine feminine" would have seemed a little out-there to most—and I was in England, not California, after all. Logic, linear thinking, and an attitude of "keep calm and carry on" was very much the name of the game.

But there's a funny thing about being pregnant. It will shake you up like no other experience if you let it, turning your normal ways of doing things on their head and opening a door into a part of you that hasn't yet spoken. Perhaps it's because all of a sudden, you are making choices for two people, not one—your inner mama lion wakes up to fight for another more than she might ever for herself. Or perhaps it starts even before that selflessness kicks in. What pregnant woman hasn't felt her senses becoming super sharp as previously benign smells, tastes, or even sounds become grating? My theory is that when you're pregnant, all kinds of things that you tolerated before—including other people telling you what to do and how and when to do them—can start to be intolerable.

Many sages, including my wizard-like aunties, say that a pregnant woman is extremely porous, able to receive insights and wisdom she previously was dulled to. They say her heightened sensitivity is her intuitive sixth sense, and is indeed her very spiritual nature waking up, sometimes dramatically. As her physical body expands, so do her sensory abilities, including, sometimes, her ability to pick up other peoples' energies (thus, her ability to connect with the spirit of her baby). As Ulrike Remlein, a womb healer and red tent facilitator who contributes her wisdom to our books, describes it, "Pregnancy more than anything else will take away the veils to the unseen world and turn you inwards." If you're ready for it, it can be your invitation to listen in deeply to what you really want and act more radically than you otherwise would.

In talking to women about their pregnancies, we found that so many will share a moment when the plan of how they assume they will "do" their pregnancy gets turned upside down. A neighbor shares her surprising birth experience; a gifted book opens to a page about doulas; an Instagram feed reveals an image of orgasmic birth. There's something about the magic of pregnancy and birth that invites in glorious disruption to your previous plans.

In my case, that disruption came via a friend named Khefri Riley. Khefri was (and still is!) a head-turning woman—an artist and activist who sparkles with Shakti. To me, a quasi-tomboy who'd grown up in the orbit of my slightly older brother Hsuan, she was like some kind of cosmic mermaid. Khefri had become pregnant two years before me, and the artist in her drove her to bolder-than-average choices, seeking out a water birth at a birth center (still quite uncommon at the time) and prenatal Kundalini yoga. Though I didn't know it then, Khefri's passion had been stoked by her connection to her ancestors, who were Afro-Indigenous grandmother midwives in the American South. Black Grand Midwives of the South cared for mothers-to-be and "caught" countless babies in the years before birth became medicalized, taken out of the home and out of the hands of traditional Black birth workers and the communities they served. These heroic Black women were anchor points of their communities, holding the health and safety of both Black and white mothers in their hands. They also kept the knowledge of local plant medicines as well as the most private and intimate stories of the community—as her father would say, "They were legendary!" Khefri's great-grandmother, her grandmother, and even her father, who (in his youth) held the oil lanterns for these women as they worked at night, passed on to her what she referred to as "the sacred flame of womb wisdom." And then she passed that flame to me.

Through a series of very non-logical (but very intuitive!) steps, I charted a course back to my former hometown of Los Angeles with my then-husband, six months pregnant and without proper health insurance. (Chalk that part up to being an artsy, globe-trotting twentysomething.) Like some kind of super focused homing pigeon, I found my way to a highly seasoned Sikh midwife named Davi Kaur Khalsa who had space for me in her practice and—miraculously—took Medi-Cal. Davi became my beloved prenatal care provider, breathtakingly skilled in handling the science and medicine side of healthy gestation and safe delivery. She taught all the mothers under her care that when four pillars were in place—eating well, daily walking (a lot of it, the bigger you got), gentle yoga or stretching to stay limber and aligned in the spine and pelvis, and some kind of quiet time or meditation to stay calm and connected to themselves—the vast majority of pregnancies and deliveries were healthful and positive experiences. She also became something else: my first mentor in the sweet, tender, and enriching art of pregnancy. By that, I mean the complement to the science and biology part of it all—the private and more inward-facing way of moving through the journey that each person practices in their own very personal way. Walking into Davi's softly lit, beautifully decorated midwifery center, taking my shoes off, and receiving her generous hug of greeting as melodious music played softly in the background, my nervous system got the message: Slow down and settle in; it's time to connect with how you're feeling and share everything that's going on. An exhale of relief swept through me at every visit as years of unspoken tension held in my body softened, releasing into this safe and unconditionally loving container.

Looking back now, I realize how tough I'd been at that age, embarking on the path to motherhood without my own mother at my side, or any maternal figures in my life. It's how a lot of us enter into mothering—emboldened and independent, but oddly untethered to those who've done it before. Becoming mothers without mothers to mother us is a bit like being a solitary astronaut heading bravely to the moon. I most certainly wouldn't have been able to articulate it then—I was shut down about this kind of stuff, in part due to sexual abuse I'd experienced at home and the boundaries and distance I'd installed for my well-being—but I see it now. It's the invisible element of parenting we just don't talk about much in our society but that contributes to making it easier: the encircling presence of others who've succeeded in walking the path before you, and wholeheartedly believe that you can do it too.

Perhaps that is what the ember had actually lit up—a very ancient and persistent desire I hadn't known existed: I want to feel encircled! How blessed I am that Davi and my friend Khefri—who'd become, magically enough, a trained doula as her ancestors had practically ordained—became my first small circle of maternal supporters. I plugged into their power and belief in me when I delivered my first daughter—whom I named Khefri in honor of this bond—and plugged into these powerhouses again for my second and third births, letting their belief affirm and intensify my own self-trust as I delivered my children India and Jude. Each time, as I grew in confidence and willingness to use my voice, my birthing circle of support got a little bigger. (By my third birth, two friends and their baby arrived before the placenta was delivered, to lovingly cheer me on.) For each one, I envisioned, then mentally sketched out, the conditions that my instincts told me worked best for me. These primal, powerful experiences of giving birth were my masterpieces! And I held them close like a talisman, reminding me in some tough times that followed of just how capable and worthy I was. After years of being in awe of the human body's ability to grow life and birth, that awe became personal: my own body working according to its incredible design. I'd always slightly questioned the value of my femaleness and hovered slightly outside my own body as a result. But after birthing my children, those questions evaporated. The long-frozen parts of myself—my relationship to my physique, my emotions, and my senses— began to thaw.

My three pregnancy and birthing experiences gifted me with several things: an undying awe for the profound work that birthkeepers do, a keen awareness of the way one woman ignites a spark in the next to reach for more out of her pregnancy, and a deep love of the culture and community of pregnancy and mother care. Because what so often gets lost in our focus on the outward-facing parts of pregnancy—all the choices we must make and actions we must take, all the information we must sort through and forms to fill out—is the quieter truth that motherhood is a communal experience. While women can certainly carry off tremendous things on our own—and so often, we have to do it that way—most every part of it goes better when we have each other at our sides.

To me, trusting in companions who believe in you and are there for you feels like trusting in nature. There is a sense that—in one pocket of your life at least— things are in the right order. And it's amazing how when that sense of rightness is in place, you are liberated to find out just how much you have within yourself. Mama Khefri (as my daughter now calls her) said it best when, a good twenty years after we first met and in reminiscence for this book, she told me, "Birth is the final frontier of liberating the body because the body holds so much wisdom innately within us. It teaches us that nobody has to give it to us and we don't have to go anywhere for it. We have it within ourselves."

––––––––––––––

A couple of years after Jude was born, I started to cook postpartum meals professionally for mothers in Los Angeles, inspired by what the Chinese medicine practitioners in my family had taught me about the crucial importance of dedicated and nurturing postpartum care. Hybridizing the ancient art of *zuo yuezi* (or "sitting the month") for a new audience caught on, our book *The First Forty Days* came out, and suddenly my circle grew much bigger. I was plugged into a veritable cosmos of bold, fierce, tender, and capable maternal supporters, from midwives to labor and delivery nurses, and from doulas to OBs—and acupuncturists, pelvic floor healers, energy workers, therapists, and everything in between—all dedicated to accompanying women through their pregnancy journeys. As a one-time oddball outcast—the birth nerd lost in reverie on the bookstore floor!—I'd finally found my tribe.

The more I have explored these galaxies of care, the more respect I've gained for what the pregnancy experience can be. It is not just an in-between phase of your life (between the state of not having a child and having one) but a challenging, profound, and transformational one in and of itself.

Becoming a mother almost always breaks open a part of yourself you haven't yet explored. I've heard versions of this many times over and over while feeding

> To see the power and intensity coming from a woman fully committed to her own growth is beautiful. It is challenging to do the work from girl to mother in the labor space. The journey must begin prenatally.
>
> —HAIZE HAWKE, *master doula and advanced primary midwife student*

moms my MotherBees meals. A woman who considered herself deeply practical and no nonsense before giving birth gets lost in oxytocin-soaked head nuzzling, all other responsibilities be darned. A wishy-washy type digs in her heels and gets grounded as she's forced to bring organization and structure into her life with an infant. A self-centered diva—yes, some will admit to being one of those!—finds the part of her that is pure devotion and service. No matter which way the delivery of your child looks—assisted or unassisted, vaginal or cesarean—the process asks you to completely let go of one version of yourself and birth the next version. Mythologically speaking, it's a transition from wide-eyed Maiden—full of wonder, yet still girlish, the inner roar untapped—to full-on Mother, on fire with a capability that's never burned so hotly before.

Some psychologists dub pregnancy a "crisis." What they mean is that it is a unique developmental phase in a woman's life where she encounters the unknown, tests her fortitude and trust, goes through a climax point—a peak experience—that pushes her to plumb her most-hidden depths, and then digests the experience (during the postpartum phase), gradually integrating or making sense of her new identity of Mother (or Mother Again). Intense as it sounds—and it is!—this crisis is by design a positive upheaval, a turning point of self-discovery and realization. Or at least it can be, if the process is recognized as meaningful and given appropriate space, time, and support to occur.

How disappointing, then, that for so many women, that is far from what they receive. Ask mothers who've recently given birth if they truly felt seen, held, and heard during their pregnancy, and acknowledged for the scale, complexity, and specialness of what they're doing, and the answers will be very diverse. A significant number will say the attention and care they received while pregnant—primarily in the form of prenatal visits as well as the professional care received during the birth itself—seemed adequate or satisfactory, if a little impersonal. Many others report feeling shunted through a system that they didn't quite understand, or that was never adequately explained. Some percentage of both these groups—a much larger number of people than we collectively want to acknowledge—wrestle with experiences that hindered, hurt, or even traumatized them or made them feel sidelined or shut up. Of course, many women are telling a brighter story—that they felt warmly cared for, personally witnessed, and lovingly empowered throughout. A small fraction are even taking matters firmly into their own hands, stepping radically outside current convention and designing their own care protocols or free birthing. It's the modern-day pregnancy polarity at play: The industry of pregnancy and birth is, in many countries, ratcheting up medical interventions to ever-higher levels and speeding patients through care. Yet the culture of pregnancy and birth at large is also being permeated by the influence of the gentler, kinder midwife model of care (MMOC), with its more holistic and individualized approach to mother-baby well-being. We are standing in a both/and moment, finding our feet in it, and inviting each person to figure out what they want, what they can reach for, and what they are willing to fight for too.

We're starting to talk about this polarity when it comes to the public side of pregnancy. (I still remember witnessing the reaction to my friends Ricki Lake and Abby Epstein's groundbreaking film, *The Business of Being Born*—it was major!) Long-held assumptions and intractable-seeming systems are starting to be confronted, especially about the intersection of our health care and insurance systems with socioeconomic factors and, very significantly, the implicit and explicit biases experienced during prenatal care, labor and delivery care, and postpartum care by mothers of color. The fact that Black women in the US are several times more likely to die in or after childbirth than white women, and that physical complications and psychological impacts are unforgivably higher as well, is finally landing in the public consciousness. A much-needed movement for change is beginning to rise.

But the availability and access to meaningful support is rarely discussed when it comes to a woman's private milieu. We're not yet having the quiet reckoning we need about whether a mother-to-be receives the time, space, and acknowledgment she truly needs at home, at work, in her community, and in her life at large. This lack, whether it is compounded by under-respectful or under-resourced prenatal health care, is surprisingly universal. As my friend, the doula and wellness empowerment coach Lori Bregman, told me, "Birthing people are not getting the support they need, and they don't just need information. They need support to make their own good choices." While this dilemma has gotten worse in the extraordinary circumstances under which we are writing this book—the COVID pandemic that has made care visits even shorter and harder to get and evaporated physical touch and intimate contact for many expecting mothers—it is highlighting weaknesses that have been there for decades.

And when a pregnant woman is under-supported—when there is a gap between what she needs and what she gets—these weaknesses can become gaping holes. If others don't recognize the woman's need for quality rest, the opportunity for daily stress management, and the consistent, well-balanced nutrition that her rapidly changing body deserves, gestational health issues can arise that might otherwise not. Without guidance into the type of professional support she deserves, and help in sourcing it and then, critically, advocating for her right to have it, situations can arise around labor and delivery that put her body and her baby in jeopardy— very often, unnecessarily so. For women whose families have their own indigenous traditions of maternal care, the effect of having that support totally left out of the room, as is most often the case today, can be wrenching and disorienting.

Less obviously, but equally as important, when society-at-large expects an expecting mother to pull off everything she pulled off before (and then some, most likely), and offers her few concessions of extra space and time, it can starve her of the chance to prepare physically and mentally for giving birth—one of the most intense initiations she will likely ever go through. That's not good. When a woman feels rushed, stressed, resistant, or scared, labor and delivery can bring a level of complication it might not otherwise bring.

The Modern Pregnancy Support Gap

The pitfalls of the under-supported pregnancy journey are real. When generous, mother-centered care is unavailable, it feeds into a plethora of often unnecessary problems. Today we are seeing surging levels of largely avoidable pregnancy complications like gestational diabetes and preeclampsia; skyrocketing medical interventions during labor and delivery that, while life-saving when indicated, can also be traumatizing when not; and high rates of postpartum challenges like anxiety and depression. Not to mention new motherhood hurdles like exhaustion, sleep disturbance, and even the onset of autoimmune disease triggered by pregnancy. All this contributes to an epidemic of maternal and familial strain that is under-discussed but prevalent; mothers operating without enough backup feel torn as finite reserves of energy become insufficient to meet every need. Co-parents and partners feel it equally—plus the lack of their partner's full presence. Now add a bow on it: In the US, all this is compounded by a historically egregious lack in prenatal and postpartum maternal and paternal paid leave or social support. Meanwhile, as pressures mount, instead of receiving more understanding and practical help—the kind that meets women where they are—they're more likely to be bombarded with advice and information about how they could be doing it all better. No wonder the modern-day motherhood experience is not nearly as soft and fuzzy as greeting cards and diaper ads would have us believe! Anger and grief around unexpected curveballs, and disappointment around experiences missed, can be as common a sentiment as giddy, rose-toned joy. In my conversations with OBs and labor and delivery nurses, I know that many of them feel likewise—their progressive instincts can get hampered by the system's grip and liability concerns. It's a pickle! But what changes might ripple outward to improve the mothering experience at large if we bridged this gap from the very outset and ensured that the pregnancy journey was better supported and less prone to cracks and failings?

The support gap can also contribute to hidden hairline cracks that, if left unaddressed, can start to cause fractures in relationships with others or even within the mother's own psyche. Most mothers are happy to receive thoughtful care for the growing baby in their belly. But they may not know their own inner growth—less visible, less trackable than the baby's—is spectacularly special and deserves thoughtful attention as well. After all, in this time of mind-blowing fetal growth and development, the mother is also reorganizing herself, going from Maiden to Mother or Mother Again and upgrading her identity and purpose—that's no small psychic overhaul! But when society at large acts blasé about it—barely acknowledging this may be happening or turning a glazed eye to her request to be given a break—it can create, at best, an odd disconnect between her reality and that of the world at large, and, at worst, a crisis not of the good kind.

> In modern pregnancy there is a lot of fear-mongering. It's all about prohibitions, when really it should be about replenishing.
>
> —SABINE WILMS, *historian of Chinese medicine*

As our photographer Jenny McNulty described, nine months pregnant with her first baby and with two young stepchildren at her feet, "I feel guilty saying, 'I need quiet time and peace at home; and I also need support and company now from my friends.'" She described an acute awareness of the vulnerability that (no surprise here) had kicked in as her body got bigger, slower, and a little less agile, and as the reality of what was coming drove an instinctual need to be held close—even clingily so at times—by her partner and loved ones. "I don't feel I can ask for help before my due date, when baby is here for all to see."

It's not surprising that when mothers share their pregnancy stories in a safe, supported space, tears can come and there's a choke in the throat, even years after the events they are describing. For every woman who's had a juicy, inspired, and empowering pregnancy and birth experience, there are quite a few more who have felt overly alone, fearful, or stretched thin.

As Davi once told me, being pregnant isn't easy in America.

A Precious Legacy

Over the years of providing meals for new mothers (and spreading the word about postpartum care in our books), I have watched in awe as women around the globe have started to claim a period of dedicated rest and recovery after their baby is born. They've asked partners and friends to take responsibilities off their shoulders and have rewritten the script around what new mothers should be asked to do. It's hard to capture how good it is to feel the force of women putting their own needs first.

Yet when I began to expand my MotherBees reach by creating meals specially for the pregnancy phase, designed to ensure a mother-to-be was as vital, supported, and cared for as can be, an interesting thing happened at first. Nothing. Women didn't take me up on the offer! "Sure," they seemed to be saying, "We'll take support and nurturing after we've produced the goods, but while all's still under wraps, I don't deserve the help." How counterintuitive! The pregnant person is only building, housing, and feeding another human, all from her very cells and tissues, and developing their brain with her nutrients and helping make their hormones and immune system, month after month, all the while experiencing a gamut of her own odd bodily sensations, moments of genuine discomfort, and possible sleep disturbances, while also holding down all her regular duties at home or at work. She's also preparing (or totally overhauling) the home front for what's to come and caring even more ardently than ever for others (other children, pets, and yes, her partner or spouse!) knowing they'll soon be eclipsed by a baby. What extra help could she possibly need?

When I was inducted into my elders' traditions of postpartum care at the end of my first pregnancy, it was an aha moment about the amplifying effects of giving birth. In the old ways that my relatives knew about, gestating and delivering a baby is one of three portals a woman walks through in her life. These portals are profound opportunities for either consolidating and strengthening her vitality, resiliency, and beauty, or weakening and depleting them. (The pregnancy portal is the second of them; the first is the onset of fertility at adolescence, and the third is the onset of menopause.) So crucial is the pregnancy and postpartum portal that, in the two-and-a-half-thousand-year-old tradition of *yang sheng*—China's venerated science of nourishing life that we might call, less romantically, preventive health care—the level of care a woman experiences in this time is considered as influential over her total lifetime as the more obvious pillars like good diet, quality sleep, and regular exercise. In fact, the lifestyle she follows, nourishment she receives, and mental and emotional balance she maintains as she moves

> A peaceful and healthy pregnancy may help a woman recover from a long-standing disease, while a pregnancy disturbed by poor nutrition, emotional trauma, and stress can impact negatively on her health for years to come.
>
> —PETER DEADMAN, *Live Well Live Long: Teachings from the Chinese Nourishment of Life Tradition*

through her pregnancy greatly influence the outcome of each life-changing portal and color how smoothly she moves into the next portal and through the remainder of her life. There is recognition that, as she moves through these three doorways, her body is in massive transition—changing, evolving, refining, establishing new cycles, or letting old ones go. They are moments of great opportunity and vulnerability. Of the three, pregnancy has the biggest amplification effect on her current state of well-being: The old ways take very seriously any cracks in the foundation at this time, and very notably in the recovery weeks after giving birth. Poor diet, overexertion or lack of rest, or sudden shock or trauma that occurs during pregnancy can cause a ripple effect of disorder or even disease, and will take deliberate and thoughtful care to resolve. For this reason, the personalized care received during all phases of pregnancy and birth is so important that it's engrained as a non-negotiable in many families in China. (One statistic says that 30 percent of the almost $100 billion home care industry there is devoted to mother-child care!) There is a very real recognition that childbearing is a very draining process on a woman's body, and it's understood that not receiving help does not spare others trouble or time. Instead, it creates a debt that can, if not paid off, lead to depletion, depression, or disconnect from self, baby, or partner.

When I began looking deeper into my own heritage of maternal care, seeking to know how women were cared for holistically, and through food in the past, I was profoundly moved by just how long this recognition has existed. Even as far back as the fourth century BCE, the classic texts of Chinese medicine conferred eminent status to a woman's reproductive health. Wise one Sabine Wilms, a new friend and a historian of Chinese medicine, shared with me how the thinker Sun Simiao, in his seventh century encyclopedia of health, rather wonderfully titled *Essential Prescriptions for Every Emergency Worth a Thousand in Gold*, places gynecology first before all other concerns. Sabine says, "The woman is seen as the foundation of health. Looking at the practitioners of the tenth, eleventh, and twelfth centuries, there is an incredibly sophisticated understanding of women's health that I would argue is far superior to any Western biomedicine doctor today. The ancient texts contain so much information about preparing for pregnancy, and attuning the menstrual cycle to the lunar and cosmic cycles."

A kindred historian, Nicole Richardson, described to me how in the ancient traditions of China, the mother was seen to have cosmological significance. "All of creation depends on her, and there is a lot of power in her role—she raises the next generation of the lineage." In a worldview that did not see separation between humans and nature, a remarkably holistic approach to mother and fetus took hold. Millennia before Western science cottoned on, Chinese medicine looked deeply at the ways the mother's health, well-being, and emotional state (which in turn were shaped by external influences) influenced the baby's development in utero. They even laid out protocols around diet and activity, comportment, and mindset, to avoid pregnancy complications and to create harmony within and around the mother. Called *taijiao*, which translates to fetal education or, more properly, fetal cultivation, these guidelines and taboos were said to help ensure a physically and morally upstanding offspring. Listening to harmonious music, eating appropriate flavors, avoiding salacious or disturbing imagery, and cultivating peace of mind were encouraged—if not outright prescribed—and modifications from one trimester to the next reflected the mother's changing needs. From an inward-oriented and protected first trimester to prevent the dangers of disordered chi, to a fortifying and satiating second trimester (when "it is appropriate for her to eat the meat of birds of prey and wild beasts," according to Sun Simiao), the instructions culminate in a third trimester reveling in ripeness, when, as Sabine told me, "the mom loosens her belt, lets her hair down, gets spoiled and served sweet wine, and is all about letting go!"

When I learned about this, I couldn't help but picture my great-great-grandfather Dr. Huang, a beloved member of his community, sitting amongst jars of herbs in his long-ago practice. I wondered (my full birth nerd, artistic reverie kicking in), would he have dispensed advice to a pregnant one about munching on meat of prey, or looking calmly at lotus flowers? Of course, from a contemporary perspective, being instructed to read poetry to your belly or even to practice good posture—because it will create an upstanding child, according to Simiao—can smack of just a tad oppressive. (Though it's certainly an intriguing idea to "handle objects made of white jade and observe peacocks" to guarantee a beautiful baby!) We don't have a direct line back to ask women of yore how they felt about it, nor first-person written accounts from mothers and matriarchs of their experience. Yet even with these queries, I can't help but be awed by this artful, early recognition of all the ways a pregnant woman's mind and body are connected to her environment. Acknowledging how her sensory perceptions of the world filter inward to her womb and how her needs morph in an ever-changing, cyclical flow is a far cry from dismissing (or downright ignoring) the subtle fields of thought and emotion, as many report about their prenatal care today! Romanticized or not, in my mind's eye, the old teachings seem to hold the mother in an elevated place, floating as if on a soft, radiant cloud. How moving that, centuries ago, the mother-to-be was given such a treasured status—never sidelined—and allowed to exist, well fed, well rested, and peaceful in the center of it all, aglow with vitality like the sun.

Deeply Deserving of Care

What inspires me most from my ancestral teachings on childbearing—the part that feels more relevant for today—is how deeply a pregnant woman deserves a special space of support and a dedicated circle of care. Though not, in my opinion, because it helps her bear virtuous and morally straight offspring for the honor of the family line. (Though that's a nice side effect, to be sure!) To me—and to so many of the birthkeepers and pregnancy experts I have met—these things matter because they gift a mother-to-be with the opportunity to fully sink into her pregnancy in a way that supports her safety and mental and emotional well-being, and that awakens pleasure and self-pride. Less rushed, less burdened, she can transit more gradually and deliberately through it (even through the bumpy and uncomfortable parts, of which there are likely to be a few). With her mental bandwidth less jammed by noise, she is more able to tune in to her needs, dreams, and wants. Better resourced and rested as a result, she can have the strength to voice those desires. While none of this guarantees a perfect, painless physical birth outcome, these things almost always ensure that, holistically speaking, the transition into Mother (or Mother Again) goes smoother than it might otherwise. Just as it's often said that a woman in labor does best when allowed to fully be in the process, deeply connected to herself, and undisturbed by unnecessary intrusion or disruption, one can make the strong case that it's the same with pregnancy as a whole.

But holding space for this sinking in feels like something of a lost art today! Rather than safeguarding women against depletion and shoring up cracks with deep care before, during, and after pregnancy, we push them past reasonable limits. Rather than allowing them leeway to make sense of this crossing and get familiar with the strange new landscape ahead, we barely acknowledge they're moving anywhere new at all. And far from slowly, deliberately ramping up to that threshold moment of delivering a child—taking care to fill the reserves, counsel the psyche, and assure the spirit—we slingshot the pregnant person across it, expecting them to stick the landing while deftly holding a newborn, with a picture-ready smile to boot.

Frustratingly, as a society we've come to expect that the expecting woman doesn't need much of anything special at all.

Since my very first encounter with my midwife Davi Khalsa, when I walked into her cozy, womblike treatment rooms, I've held close the vision of a soft and cushy space of retreat for every pregnant person. When I was a little girl, fascinated by round-bellied mamas-to-be, I used to imagine rolling out a red carpet before their feet, in honor of their sacred state. Once I became pregnant myself, that red carpet became more like a rose-toned sanctum in my mind, stocked with blankets, pillows, and lavender scents—a supersensory and nurturing "room of her own," where a mother could rest, expand, open little by little, and, radiant as a flower, exude her golden glow. And so I started to wonder, as I cooked my MotherBees soups and brewed teas for women before, during, and after their childbearing experience: Given the demands, rush, and burdens put on so many pregnant women today, what would it look and feel like to occupy a space like that? Could we reclaim some of that artful care of the past and help a woman sink into her pregnancy experience with a sigh of contentment and relief?

I knew the feeling I wanted to offer to her—a feeling of being truly held, seen, and valued to her core—but I didn't know how to arrive at it. So I began asking others.

> The amount of information we have today is so overwhelming. It sometimes just separates a woman from who she is. So let her go back to simple things, and connect with her roots.
>
> —DAVI KAUR KHALSA, *midwife*

Amely, Marisa, and I began plugging into our birthing cosmos: the global, wide-reaching circle of wise ones who generously contribute to our books. These experts carry the art of caring for women in their very essence, after holding, rocking, empowering, and protecting them through all of their personal portals, cumulatively many, many times over. Truth be told, we think of these profound and deeply connected people as our Crones—the keepers of the deep knowledge of the woman's journey. (Mythologically, the Crone is the third of the three archetypes of the woman's life journey, after Maiden and Mother.) We wondered if they'd deliver to us some kind of legendary handbook handed down from the past, a reliable guide to artful and meaningful pregnancy care. But such is the unpredictable nature of pregnancy, in which best laid intentions often go belly up: There wasn't one! Instead, our Crones offered us strand after strand of unstructured wisdom, adding up to a fabric of mothering that was more forgiving, more allowing, and more intuitive than any to-do list could be. Over hours of conversation with them in India and Germany and Indonesia and California, as they shared their knowledge, we began to see common themes in their advice; we found four simple, universal insights that were beautifully and quite movingly ordinary.

1

Treat Yourself Gently

The old ways of Chinese medicine have the pregnant person firmly held in social networks, with others in the family tending closely to her care. It's likewise in the millennia-old science of life from India known as Ayurveda. Dr. Padma Raju, a reputed *vaidya* (doctor) from the highly esteemed Raju family of practitioners, shared how in her tradition, the expecting mother is pampered by older women in her family and community from the day of conception until weeks after delivery. Everyone helps ensure she is well fed in order to build her reserves while soothing and grounding her nerves, and helping keep anxiety and stress at bay. Padma, along with all of our wise ones, insists that a mother-to-be is never left to fend for herself.

In Indonesia, Ibu Robin Lim, one of our heroes and founder of the Bali-based community health, education, and childbirth center Bumi Sehat Foundation, and the granddaughter of a midwife and healer herself, passionately advocates for a "continuum of woman-to-woman care" in pregnancy that supports a mother's sense of safety and spiritual reassurance. "Gentle landings and first embrace, these are all what women do for each other." Robin is the author of one of my favorite pregnancy books, *The Ecology of Gentle Birth*, and in her world, a mother-to-be barely even has to say what she needs; those around her are so attuned to anticipating her needs, allowing her to truly just be. How different it is from our modern Western tough-it-out mentality in which competency and consistency are prized, and vulnerability is—no bones about it—avoided or even outright feared! It's more common to aim for superheroine status, folding pregnancy into an already full load, rather than risk looking weak or needy. The older ways teach that the "what doesn't kill you makes you stronger" mentality, while valuable for many endeavors in life, is not appropriate for pregnancy, a time when a woman should have full permission to ask for help. And there's a sublime silver lining to doing it. Says Dr. Padma, "When a woman is properly taken care of and nourished in pregnancy, the child will be very awake, very intelligent, very spiritual—I have seen this over and over!"

2

Buffer the Worry

The old ways teach that with all the changes occurring in the body, the normal balance in the mind is more likely to be disturbed. Ayurveda credits this to the surge in *vata* that occurs as a new human is being grown. Vata, the biological force (or *dosha*) of creation, is associated with movement and air, and when it is heightened, anxious and restless thoughts as well as feelings of loneliness or low spirits are quite naturally at play, just as winds blow in the spring. Similarly, the ancient taijiao teachings put keeping a peaceful heart and mind as paramount in importance. Anticipating that unsettled feelings are a quite normal phenomenon helps a mother-to-be layer in soft buffers against anxiety as well as loneliness or negativity before it begins, and not get taken by surprise. Dr. Padma shares how these can be all sorts of things, from movement and breathing practices to calm the nervous system; to reading or hearing uplifting—or even mythological—stories of pregnancy, mothering, and birth; to the most obvious of all: drawing close those people who bolster you with positive energy. Again, that asking-for-help thing rears its head. Says Padma, "It's the responsibility of whoever is around the woman to ensure

> Understanding that chaos can exist outside of me but peace and calmness can also exist inside me is not only good for the mother, it is a boon to the baby for all his life.
>
> —DAVI KAUR KHALSA

she is occupied and does not feel lonely." This doesn't have to mean grand gestures. Little ones, like frequent companionship and light, or hopeful conversations about all the good to come, help calm any agitation and give the pregnant person more comfort than the giver may even know.

3

Surround Yourself with Sweetness

As I'll reiterate in the Feed Yourself Well chapter, we're not talking about mainlining sugar here. Rather, we are feeding the senses with beauty and feeding the heart with love, just as intentionally as feeding the cells with good nutrition. You may certainly gaze at peacocks and white jade like my predecessors if you like— or sensuous plants or gorgeous flowers!—but know that sweetness is found in quite simple gestures too. Ibu Robin Lim celebrates "the daily rituals that women do for each other, like giving prayers over the food, or even just centering yourselves for a moment, to make sure what the mother eats is lovely and nourishing." Dr. Padma shares how filling the home with "soft and smooth" music brings purity and positivity into the milieu, and how taking special herbal baths helps uplift the expecting one's spirits. While the ancient Chinese practices teach that in the first trimester exposure to beautiful art, music, or words actually feeds into how well the fetus develops its physical form, we might more easily connect to the ways these things affect the mother's state of being. Enjoying the colors and textures of the clothes you wear, pausing to feel moved by a verse of song or a favorite chapter in a book, or delighting in the prettiness of foods on your plate or the artfulness of the cup in your hand all create harmony between mind and heart. This inner cohesiveness can also spill over into blissful togetherness between mother and child. And let's not forget the cherishing sensation of touch. My friend, the late Chumash medicine woman Cecilia Garcia, used to reflect that those in the mother's intimate circle should touch her and stroke her hair sweetly, literally putting love into her with their hands. As Dr. Padma sees it, "Love gives more strength to the woman; even if just from one person, if they are giving enough love and enough care, that is more than enough for the woman to grow in confidence and strength. She will develop more of both from that love."

4

Claim Your Crown

The texts of Ayurveda teach that "the aura of a pregnant woman is one of the easiest to see, for it is particularly luminous and full of gold." No wonder that in subtler traditions, the mother-to-be is honored for what she is creating and contributing to the whole! There's a splendor to this endeavor, and being recognized for it doesn't have to wait until the little one is here: The spiritual significance of becoming a mother is worthy of its own honoring. At key points during the pregnancy, Ayurveda celebrates her almost as a goddess whose work of bringing a new soul into the world is honored with adornments, silks, and gifts (with just a touch of cardamom-infused candy). For Robin Lim, recognizing the spiritual significance of pregnancy is as critical to a mother's care as respect for science and for nature. "In Bali, *adot* means 'spirit'; what makes you spiritually safe," Robin says. "That, to us, is the most important. When a woman feels spiritually supported, as well as nutritionally supported, she finds success in gentle pregnancy and birth." This feeds in to what Robin sees as the meta-meaning of the entire pregnancy, birth, and mothering experience: "To awaken your inner knowing." For Robin, pregnancy offers a grand unfolding, a golden opportunity to know more of who you are.

> Unfolding as a mother will help you get in touch with your awake and wonderful inner knowing.
>
> —IBU ROBIN LIM, *midwife*

Our Crones (including our honorary male contributor, Damian Hagglund) told us not to be deceived by the simplicity of what they shared. These insights are not just throwaway strands of advice; they are robust braids, things you can hold on to. And when an expecting one does so, she can flourish. She can be better tethered to the experience—less apt to get lost in overwhelm or unmoored by all the change. She is less likely to fall into the trap of overgiving, which can lead to a habit of self-sacrifice, or even abandoning herself. And most simply and perhaps most profoundly of all, she can feel sure of her inner capabilities, even if the perfect outer conditions—like having the ideal care team around her or a birth plan followed to the T—don't manifest, or aren't within reach in the first place.

Together, these four insights offered a suggestion of how to practice the art of pregnancy—the private, personal, and inward complement to the linear science of it all. The next question my cowriters and I faced was how to do that art. How could a pregnant person, or one who hopes to become pregnant, and those who are supporting the pregnant ones, create an enriched, cared for, and personally meaningful pregnancy experience today?

Putting It into Practice

There's a high chance your pregnancy landscape does not feature a grandmother ladling warm soup into your bowl or aunties adorning you with silks and gold. It's likely that your employer would balk at letting you sink into a restful cocoon of care for forty weeks (even if they might honor the forty days after baby is born). And friends may be gung ho to throw a shower for baby and a blessingway for you further down the line—that's the fun part, after all!—but their calendars may be filled up in months one through nine. Furthermore, if you're like many women in the US, your access to even basic care may be unforgivably complicated or limited, through no fault of your own. It just isn't realistic for most pregnant people to re-create an entire social network oriented to their deep and devoted care.

But it is possible to weave a small net of support for yourself—a net of care that is so personal that maybe only you can see or know it is there, like a delicate but strong web that holds you a bit, letting you sink more easefully into the experience of gestating and delivering a child. As we began to gather up all the insights, rituals, and practices our wise ones shared about creating a more golden pregnancy experience—one infused with softness, support, and a sense of being seen, heard, and valued—we also pulled in the honest sharings of new mothers in our circles, and we even went through our own intimate reminiscences. We captured the voices, thoughts, visions, and hopes of those who have walked this path many times before and those who are still on it, or have very freshly come off it. Weaving them all together, we realized we had a basket of offerings for a pregnant person to pick through and use as she likes—small gifts that help her practice a very personalized art of pregnancy care throughout her forty weeks.

Sitting in the center of the basket, of course, is food. For me, making nourishing and visually beautiful food is the most tangible way of practicing self-care and responding to the shifting needs of body, mind, and heart. We eat daily—in some way or form, at least—and while pregnancy brings unique challenges, such as losing the love of food completely for days (or weeks) at a time, or finding once-favorite treats temporarily repellent (or totally indigestible), cooking and preparing food remains the epicenter of self-love for me. It is the most-used brush in my life-artist kit. Preparing good food, or asking others to prepare it for you, ignites an instant shift into a state of higher self-worth, a state that I believe is at the heart of a golden pregnancy experience. (And beyond that, of a golden life as well!) To that end, you'll discover forty-seven food and beverage recipes, plus snack ideas, that are easy, friendly, and kind in spirit, and not complex or demanding in the least. Little gems that will light you up! I created them to not only feed your growing body well, but to inspire you to take a few minutes to nourish your body, delight your senses, or soothe your state of mind no matter how busy your day seems to be.

Around these colorful recipes, loosely held in our basket of offerings, are an assortment of equally precious practices, rituals, and reflections to draw you deeper into your inward-oriented experience—the part of pregnancy that nobody else can judge, approve of, or evaluate. There's no right way to use these nuggets; rather, sit with them, pick them up and look at them, and feel into what they bring up for you. Try some of the practices and reflect on some of the words shared with the same tenderness you will soon give to your child, just first turned to yourself. Move through these sections fluidly, following their flow.

For they have a movement of their own. As the three of us—myself, Marisa, and Amely—collected up these pearls of wisdom from our wise ones, they began to organize themselves into five glimmering, shining clusters—constellations of sorts:

Stillness ◆ Honor ◆ Trust ◆ Intimacy ◆ Power

Quite frankly, our breath was taken away. These five clusters held so much more than just information or advice! They were treasures—illuminating gifts of the pregnancy experience that had the potential to guide a mother on the path of unfolding exactly as Robin Lim had spoken of it, each one inviting her to unearth and bring to light precious parts of her most realized self. The magic and magnificence of pregnancy had arrived—it was definitely in the room!

Rest assured, nothing about the chapters to come is prescriptive or bossy. There is no telling you what to do or what choices to make about your pregnancy and birth. It's actually the inverse. The five treasures exist to accompany you on your own personal path, nudging you, like a few devoted friends would do, to pay attention to the whispers coming from within—and then speak up about what they're telling you to do. There's no efforting involved in the pages to come. Simply be with these gifts, and even feel the flow of them inviting you inward, offering deeper connection, and then allowing an outward expansion, opening your arms to others and then standing tall in your grand and magnificent self.

> If we were more encircled, developing strong ties within the sisterhood, then even if we didn't have the outcome we wanted, we could still fall into this soft net of support and recovery and protection.
>
> —KHEFRI RILEY, *doula and women's mentor*

What is wise to heed is that all these treasures are available for use—quite eager for your engagement, actually—from the earliest moment of pregnancy until the last. The earlier you explore them, the better, for the forty weeks (or a little more or a little less) will fly by and before you know it, there you will be, big in belly, arriving at the threshold of your next phase of life. How you land in motherhood can be greatly influenced by the small, artful things you've practiced doing inwardly along the way.

For that's what these treasures offer, in truth: practice. As my own relatives impressed on me so many years ago, tending to your well-being is an art that you practice through everyday gestures and modest rituals. A choice to put the dulling food to one side and pick the next best choice; a commitment to prioritizing rest when more activity beckons; a moment of breathing slowly to center and connect when stress hits. Nobody expects perfection about any of it, either. It's one step forward, one step back; remember, then forget, then remember again.

And to offer an extra dash of relief in an already pressure-filled experience of becoming a parent, these gifts are free. You already have them within you, as it happens. So there's no onus to acquire more stuff or do more running around in this kind of pregnancy care! There is only the invitation to dig a little, to look where maybe you'd been too busy to look before—unearthing what's been hidden inside in some cases, awaiting your excited discovery, like the capacity for quiet and the well of deep trust—and then to not postpone taking a moment devoted to yourself. Once you do that, even just once or twice or here or there, you are in it. You are practicing staying connected to yourself, listening in to your needs and wants, trusting in your own abilities, and tapping into fortitude you may never have known was there. This practice is precious, because once you're through the portal of pregnancy and firmly entrenched in parenting, these are the skills that will anchor you in all kinds of weather. They will be your go-to's as making hard choices, taking bold actions, and filling up reserves of patience become your work as a parent. Which is why we invite you to hold these five treasures close now during pregnancy, so they will never be far from hand during parenting, even when you feel you're losing your footing completely. Think of it this way: You've got forty weeks, or maybe thirty-six, or maybe forty-two to practice the art of care that will stay with you for your entire parenting career, and help you learn to never abandon yourself as you care for another—what an opportunity! If you get in the groove with it now, even in the smallest of ways, this practice will show its truest gift. It will serve you, support you, and strengthen you as a mother for the thirty-six, or forty-two, or more, years to come.

> I went into my wife's pregnancy thinking I'd pull from every bag of healer tricks I had, and it humbled me to learn sometimes you have to forget everything you think you know. We forget the essentials— the soothing food, the cuddle for the mama, the holding hands after the argument—and get so lost in technicalities!
>
> —DAMIAN HAGGLUND, *marma therapy practitioner*

Sweet Medicine

As we wove together the recipes and words for this book, testing dishes and drinking tea and conjuring stories from our lives, and our mothers' lives, and their mothers' lives too, the love I felt for the communal nature of childbearing got deeper. You see, when women gather in a safe, supported space and share their pregnancy and birthing experiences, it makes for what my friend Khefri calls sweet medicine—a tonic that comforts and boosts each one on her own path, which can even be a remedy for past pains and sorrows, lifting them from her bones. So powerful is this medicine, it might even be a balm for the women who came before us—those who never got to claim the help and healing they really needed, or who never shared their stories, or who were silenced or shamed about their reproductive stories. Most certainly, it will spill over into a better pregnancy and birthing experience for our children, and their children, and theirs.

My co-writers, our wise ones, and I believe there's never been a more import-ant time to brew this sweet medicine than today. We are at a crossroads. As more people feel the fire I once felt to reclaim a supported, safe, and enriching preg-nancy experience, we are quite literally creating a new birth culture before our very eyes. It is happening! The reclaiming of better postpartum care (and gradu-ally, of better preconception care as well) is showing us that this is so.

But so many people are still excluded from this renaissance. When it comes to becoming a mother, too much inequity, disparity, and injustice is still at work. And if this rebirth doesn't include all of us, it isn't good enough for any of us. We have to circle up harder, make our tonic more robust, and be sure to brew enough sweet medicine for all.

There is so much work to be done to better our collective birth and mothering experiences. But perhaps a small piece of this can start here, with you, reading this book. When each expecting person commits to creating a personal net of sup-port, when she practices the art of pregnancy care in the ways that work best for her, and then shares her stories about what it was like for her honestly and gener-ously, she makes an offering that lifts everyone else. She models a different way and helps others unfold in their inner knowing. She takes us all closer and closer to the place where, as Ibu Robin Lim teaches, peace really does begin in birth.

Time is speeding up. There's more to do every day. We've never done enough! These maxims are said over and again until this truth feels as solid as stone. Yet what if we didn't buy in to these perceptions for a moment and grasped these nine-and-a-half months as a golden opportunity to move through life differently? We could make pregnancy more than just a race to the finish line and, certainly, so much more than a medical event. We could restore the right order of things, where the mother's state of being is held up and protected, and she's better aided in all the doing; we could empower her to take up more space and make a ruckus if required; we could collectively celebrate what she is becoming, and then remind her, just as we are reminding you now, to pass that flame to the woman who's next in line.

THE WISE ONES

The wisdom held in these pages was born from countless conversations with the following experts. We could not have written this book without their insights and we are forever grateful for the time and energy they graciously gave to supporting this project.

LORI BREGMAN
birth doula, life coach, author, founder of Seedlyfe Superfoods
Los Angeles, California
www.loribregman.com
www.seedlyfe.com
@lbreggy

LAUREN CURTAIN
women's health acupuncturist, Chinese medicine practitioner
Victoria, Australia
www.laurencurtain.com
@laurencurtain

SIDDHI ELLINGHOVEN
spiritual guide for pregnancy, parenting, and relating
Santa Barbara, California
www.siddhisyoga.com
www.thencomesbaby.org
@siddhisyoga

MONICA FORD
fermentation specialist, founder of Real Food Devotee
Los Angeles, California
www.realfooddevotee.com
@realfooddevotee

CYNTHIA GRAHAM
health and spiritual coach
Los Angeles, California

DAMIAN HAGGLUND
marma therapy practitioner, founder of Marma Mats
New York, New York
www.marmamats.com

HAIZE HAWKE
master doula, advanced primary midwife student, board member of Temple of the Goddess, a divine feminine church
Los Angeles, California
www.haizehawke.com
@iamhaizehawkerosen

LACEY HAYNES
Co-host, *Lacey & Flynn Have Sex* podcast; founder of School of Whole and Pussy Gazing
London, United Kingdom
www.laceyandflynn.com
@laceyandflynn
@verylacey

DR. DANMEI HU, LAC
acupuncturist, founder of Healing Needle Acupuncture
Los Angeles, California

DAVI KAUR KHALSA, CNM, WHNP, MSN
certified nurse midwife, founder of TLC Woman's Center
Los Angeles, California
www.tlcwomanscenter.com

IBU ROBIN LIM, CPM
midwife, founder of Yayasan Bumi Sehat
Health Clinics
Bali, Indonesia
www.iburobin.com
www.bumisehat.org
@iburobin

YASHODA DEVI MA
master teacher of Vedic meditation and
Himalayan Yoga-Vedantic techniques for
mind/body, founder of YDM Meditation
Boulder, Colorado
www.ydmmeditation.com
@ydmmeditation

KAREN PAUL
holistic naturopath, founder of The
Source Natural Foods
Kailua, Hawaii
www.thesourcenatural.com

VAIDYA DR. PADMA NAYANI RAJU
Dr. Raju's Institute of Ayurveda
Hyderabad, India
www.drraju.com

ULRIKE REMLEIN
womb awakening mentor and red tent
facilitator
Regensburg, Germany
www.wombofjoy.com

NICOLE RICHARDSON, PHD
professor of Asian history, University of
South Carolina Upstate
Spartanburg, South Carolina
www.nicolerichardson.academia.edu

KHEFRI RILEY, CLEC, CPYT, HCHD
doula, educator, prenatal yoga specialist,
women's mysteries mentor, owner of
Los Angeles Birth Partners, codirector
of Frontline Doulas—Centering the
Community program
Los Angeles, California
www.khefri.com
www.losangelesbirthpartners.com
@soulmommagoddess
@frontlinedoulas

ROCHELLE SCHIECK
author, doula, embodied presence
facilitator, founder of Qoya Inspired
Movement
Rhinebeck, New York
www.qoya.love
@qoya.love

SABINE WILMS
historian of Chinese medicine, specialist
in medieval Chinese gynecology
Port Townsend, Washington
www.happygoatproductions.com
www.imperialtutor.com

AND MY RELATIVES
Dr. Ching Chun Ou (aka Auntie Ou),
Dr. Ju Chun Ou, Dr. Li Chun Ou, Chinese
medicine acupuncturists and herbalists
Oakland, California

THE GIFT OF

STILLNESS

GETTING PREGNANT may have been a major accomplishment, a simple process, or a surprise—however you got here, you have now gloriously arrived. You could be keeping the news tucked close to you, a secret that belongs to just you (and your partner) or you may have been sinking into this new reality for weeks, openly sharing the excitement with family and friends. Either way, there's a good chance that you are experiencing an incredibly vast range of emotions—from elation to nervousness, overwhelm to uncertainty. In a different world, and perhaps an earlier time, you would have had the space to explore these feelings, sensing how they rest in your heart, noticing how they influence your mind, and preparing mentally and emotionally for the new chapter that lies ahead. That time and space can be in short supply now.

"Being pregnant and bringing a soul into the world is the biggest job ever; yet I feel that many women don't give themselves the space to let the weight of that reality sink in," says Lauren Curtain, a women's health acupuncturist based in Victoria, Australia, who works closely with women at every stage of their reproductive journey. "It can become just something to tick off the list, before they're on to the next thing. I want to say, 'Hold it in your system for a second, tell yourself, Whoa. I fell pregnant. Wow. I'm growing a human; this is changing my life forever.'"

Lauren is a part of a growing group of birth professionals who are pointing their clients toward a richer experience of pregnancy. When a woman can access a sense of awe, wonder, or even curiosity about these forty or so weeks of gestation, pregnancy shifts from a simple process of procreation to an act of transformation. Even the smallest acknowledgment of the significance that's occurring here can help you reframe this time of your life as a precious event—the catalyst launching you into the next version of yourself where you'll step into being a Mother or Mother Again.

> I will never have this version of myself again. Let me slow down and be with her.
>
> —RUPI KAUR, *from her book* Home Body

The path to a more fulfilling pregnancy starts with a pause or a brief moment of stillness. Dare yourself to screech to a halt, or at least decrease the fervor of your pace, and you may find that you can sink into what is happening right now, touching into the full expanse of your pregnancy experience. You might even discover that it helps counter the epidemic of busyness in which many of us live. Pregnancy can offer you the gift of the present moment, where you are at least momentarily free from worry and regret—if, that is, you embrace it.

Because here's the rub: For many pregnant women, finding moments of true non-doing can be surprisingly hard. Pregnancy can be a time of go, go, go—appointments to make, milestones to meet, and gear to acquire—and that's on top, not instead, of everything else you were doing before. With no encouragement to slow down and do less, it's easy to take pride in all that you're juggling, leading you to blast through pregnancy and miss out on this incredibly potent period of your life. "With one benchmark running into the next, women often think, 'I will slow down and relax when the next milestone comes,'" Lauren explains. "Then it becomes, I'll relax when the baby arrives. But relaxation never comes—many women are simply soldiering on. It's heartbreaking."

This perpetual motion is not only exhausting, it can also take a toll. When you are caught in a web of perpetual motion, always reaching for the next goal or task to be accomplished and constantly striving, comparing, and improving, you can become constricted and uptight—a state that does not support an easeful birth and a balanced, peaceful state of mind. In this state, slowing down and finding stillness can feel even more out of reach. Until you reframe it, that is. "Society is not about stillness," doula Khefri Riley explains. "It's about external accolades and approval from others. So I ask my clients to take on the challenge of becoming still in their pregnancies so they bring the ability to find their center into their births, and then step into motherhood from a place of calm and clarity. Choosing stillness can seem *revolutionary* when the act of doing has more value than simply being."

Moving toward stillness, or at least bringing the idea to the forefront of your awareness, doesn't mean you have to let go of action, ambition, or achieving—it's more like adding a new layer to the way you have already been living. "Few women need help to *do* more in the linear, productive sense, but many of us need support in allowing ourselves to *be* more deeply," says Rochelle Schieck, founder of Qoya, a women-centric practice that has helped thousands of women access empowerment through movement. "I'm not saying one is better than the other; just that both deserve a seat at the table." If dropping down to a state of pure stillness feels like something of a leap, ramp down your expectations: Make it about simply adding some breathing room into this life-altering period of change. Imagine a small gap opening up between all the activities taking place outside of you and all the activity happening inside of you; it's in that gap that the opportunity for a more calm, vital, and empowered pregnancy resides.

The journey to stillness starts with acknowledging the need for it. Growing a baby requires a tremendous amount of energy; factoring in regular moments of rest and recharging provides an essential balance to all of that output. It may not look like it on the outside, especially in the early weeks, but gestation is an incredibly complex process with so much mysterious (almost magical!) biological action happening behind the scenes. Which makes it absolutely natural to experience extreme fatigue in the first trimester. "A lot of women feel they are being lazy because they are tired," notes Lauren. "But it can be because many of us have been conditioned to disregard inner effort. I say, 'You are growing bones right now, you are growing organs, there is so much happening internally—even if doesn't *seem* as if you are doing much, it is massive!'"

Things Are Not What They Once Were

In the early days of pregnancy, you may look like the same person to the outside world, but this is not business as usual. While you don't have to stop living your life, the first trimester does demand some notable slowing down. Historian of Chinese medicine Sabine Wilms notes that from the perspective of the ancient texts, the first three months of pregnancy are about "consolidating the fetus," creating a need for being "quiet, still, and reclusive—and avoiding alarm and fright as they disorder the vital life force known as chi." Furthermore, as your body ramps up to grow a baby, your immune system becomes temporarily suppressed as your child's immune system develops. That's why many traditional texts caution that it is easy for a pregnant woman to get sick in the early days and advise avoiding extremes of cold, heat, and wind. Many a grandmother or auntie will cluck at a pregnant one to stay warm around her core and especially her feet—the starting point for important meridians or channels of energy. To that end, accept the best seat in the house when offered; never sit casually on chilly floors, and above all, keep those tootsies warm and cozy!

When you are able to enjoy regular moments of stillness, you may begin to notice that pregnancy is made up of an intricate series of layers that are each their own universe. There are the parts of you that will be left behind when you become a Mother (or Mother Again) and the brand-new aspects of you that are preparing to rise to the surface. There will be new dynamics in your relationship with your partner, a different way of relating to how you work and play, and a massive love that is surging for this little being that you haven't met yet. With some quiet time you will find room to process all of these changes while also tracking the sea of physical sensations rolling through your body—perhaps you can even name them: tightness, tingling, or cramping. Stillness will help you notice what's happening in your body—and in your heart and mind too. This self-awareness will buoy you as you move into this next iteration of yourself, letting go of who you were and opening to the person you're becoming— someone who may feel like a stranger until you really get to know her. When taken regularly—think of it like vitamin S, a new addition to your prenatal cocktail!— stillness will forge a refuge within you that you can return to when things feel overwhelming or uncertain during pregnancy, birth, and motherhood.

> Are you really here or are you just waiting for the next thing? It's interesting to see where we are in relation to time; whether we're always between what just happened and what happens next, or whether we can be here now.
>
> —RAM DASS, *spiritual teacher and author of* Be Here Now

Getting still does not have to look a certain way. You don't need to sit in lotus position or fill a bath with rose petals (though you could do that—see Baths for a Queen, page 248). It's just about accessing what is already available. Try it now. Place this book on your lap, close your eyes, and feel its weight on your thighs. Notice the temperature of the room. Sense your clothes on your body. As you breathe normally, feel the cool air entering your nostrils and the warm air releasing. There . . . you have momentarily paused the doing. You've taken a small bite of stillness. From there, *lean into it more.* Stillness can so often lead to mindfulness and contemplation, states of mind that will hold you as you work through any fears you may have about giving birth or being a mother. It can also open the portal to letting go—a state of surrender and acceptance that will be profoundly helpful once contractions start and you are hurtling into labor with no turning back. "Look at it this way: You have nine months to prepare for giving birth, one of the most powerful letting go experiences you will ever have besides death," says Siddhi Ellinghoven. "If you practice the process of surrendering and giving over *now*, that surrender consciousness will be embedded in you by the time labor comes." If you are devouring resources about giving birth, studying the pros and cons of hypnobirthing, the Bradley method, and water birth, adding in another thing to master may sound intimidating. "But it doesn't have to be," counsels Khefri. "The question is: Can you just slow down and choose a path of nourishing yourself? All you really need is the breath. It doesn't take more than a moment of stillness and consciously choosing to do that for yourself."

Thoughtful Transitions

As you explore building moments of stillness and quiet into pregnancy, keep in mind that your environment does not have to look a certain way to offer you a slice of peace. You may find a silent pocket in unexpected places, like while sitting in your car in the driveway. Can you make it a practice to pause for a few moments before opening your car door? This creates a buffer between where you were and where you are going, and it allows you to be more present for those who will greet you in this next phase of your day. A simple break in the action can slow things down a smidge, give your body a chance to catch up with your mind, and help you drop into the present moment before racing toward the next thing. You can pause like this at any moment in the day. Try it before you turn the shower off and reach for a towel, before you bring food you've cooked to the table, or before you open the door after walking the dog.

If you find yourself resisting the act of slowing down and getting quiet, simply look down at your belly for additional motivation. Your baby will eventually be in your arms, a separate entity for you to love and care for, but today you and your baby are one. You are naturally already in a state called "entrainment"—when the rhythms and energies of two people harmonize. As such, your baby responds to, perhaps even matches, your nervous system's state. Researchers have found that babies residing in the wombs of mothers who regularly practiced Transcendental Meditation—which is similar to the technique of Vedic Meditation that several of our wise ones teach—demonstrated twice the quiet alertness of those whose mothers didn't meditate. Their nervous system is, in a sense, getting programmed to that normal of low stress and excitation. What an inspiration to bring some stress management into your everyday existence! Our spiritually minded wise ones offer added layers to this entrainment idea. Siddhi Ellinghoven, who

> Just ten minutes of stillness a day will become a woman's anchor during birth—and after it.
>
> —SIDDHI ELLINGHOVEN

has guided thousands of women through their pregnancies in her prenatal yoga classes, notes, "When an expecting mother keeps pushing to do more and more, I sense that baby feels it; the baby's soul asks, *If you don't even have time for yourself, will you have time for me?* It is a concern I have for the next generation." Yashoda Devi Ma, a teacher of time-honored Vedantic techniques for balancing body and mind, takes it further. "This child has called you to be the conveyer of their story, and *your* way of doing things may get destroyed," she explains. When you're standing at that fork in the road, wondering if you should say yes to the invitation to dinner, or to that extra task at work, or go home to rest and recharge, Yashoda suggests giving up the way you used to do things and accept the latter. "Your surrender of your preferences or old ways of being is very powerful! Surrender invokes the highest emotion of all, devotion. That's really what motherhood is about—you are devoted to another being, and to the commitment of its highest expression."

Surrendering to Challenge

So often, we fear that stressful experiences while pregnant will adversely affect our offspring. Davi Khalsa offers a new lens on this very common predicament.

"When a woman's having a particularly hard time with something that comes up during pregnancy, I say, 'This is a huge opportunity; it could be that your son or daughter came just for you to have the experience of you dealing with this challenge, so that if *they* have that challenge later in life, they'll know how to deal with it. So, let's learn how *you* can deal with it so you can teach the baby!' The truth is, life is challenging whether we like it or not; and the best thing a mother can do is to have a monkey see/monkey do approach. When she utilizes tools and techniques like meditation and breathing to stay connected to her own soul, the vibration is felt within and the baby automatically gets it. I truly believe that when their baby grows up, they will understand that they can deal with anything that erupts outside because that is not who they really are. They will know: *Me is within me.*"

In one of the beautiful paradoxes of this phase of life, pregnancy is a time to be extra gentle with yourself—and extra courageous. Letting go can feel scary. Keeping your schedule packed and your phone buzzing is a nifty avoidance

I just felt this responsibility to protect this little being. It's not only about me now; it's about this other person, and really making more time for myself in ways that felt more nourishing and allowed me to be with myself in a lot of ways. To be *with* this experience.

—AMANDA CARNEY, *new mother*

technique. When your brain is crackling with endless items to accomplish and receiving a jolt of dopamine with every ping from your device, it is easy to dodge your feelings. Now, sitting in an empty moment with some space to breathe, you may find that the fog clears and along the horizon are some very real emotions. If your path to pregnancy was challenging, with fertility hurdles or loss, pregnancy can feel especially tenuous. But even if conception was a snap, for nine-ish months you will be precariously perched between two worlds—the time before this baby and the life that comes after. Challenging feelings are a sign that there is work to be done before you move into pregnancy and motherhood. There is no better time to start than now, but don't forget to be easy on yourself. As you dip your toe into the realm of non-activity, it helps to approach this new way of being with kindness, treating yourself like you would treat a lost puppy or a frightened young child. (In Treasure Four, you will read more about what to do if anxiety or fear goes beyond mere butterflies in the tummy and requires extra support.)

Three Ways into Stillness

There are many ways to slow down and access stillness during pregnancy, but when you're revving on all cylinders, it can be tricky to find the one thing that will help you downshift. Fortunately there are a handful of simple methods that even the most type A among us can easily explore.

1

Say No

Stillness can only happen in an empty space, and to create that space, it's essential to practice saying "no." Your "no" can be to extra demands at work, social obligations, even household chores and responsibilities. You may need to take a few

SITALI PRANAYAMA

Breath Practice to Soothe Stress and Anxiety

In her prenatal yoga classes, Siddhi Ellinghoven offers this breath practice to expecting mothers experiencing stress. "With pregnancy and birth there's another feeling that gets born too," she says. "That's anxiety. We start to worry more than ever before when we become mothers, but with breath and with our fingers we can regulate our own energy, so we don't project anything onto our kids that doesn't belong to them."

This practice cleanses, strengthens, and supports the digestive system and cools and calms the body and mind. It is accompanied by the Apan Vayu mudra ("mudra" refers to a specific positioning of the fingers). This mudra is called the "lifesaver" in Indian Mudra Vigyan tradition and is designed to help with overthinking, which can lead to stress, concerns, and anxiety. The positions of the hands and tongue may seem awkward at first. It's not supposed to be pretty—don't do this one in front of a mirror!

- Sit in a comfortable cross-legged position.

- Place both hands in mudra gently on knees: bend index finger, cross the thumb over the index finger, touch tips of middle and ring fingers with tip of thumb, extend pinkie (the small intestine meridian starts at the pinkie and the heart meridian ends at the pinkie).

- Stick out your curled tongue and inhale deeply, drawing air through tongue. If you can't curl the tongue, no worries, simply purse your lips and feel the air move above your tongue as you breathe in.

- Press your tongue against the upper palate, with the tip of your tongue behind the front teeth. Close your mouth and very gently exhale through the nose.

Practice for at least three minutes, or (ideally) up to eleven minutes. Visit www.siddhisyoga.com/videos to see this and other prenatal practices.

extra steps to make "no" a reality—turning to colleagues, friends, or your partner to take up the slack. As we noted in *The First Forty Days*, when reaching out to create a support team, you will probably be surprised by how much people want to help. Chipping in gives people a chance to offer something of real value and to be part of the process—and to get those altruistic juices flowing.

"For me, one of the most empowering parts of being pregnant was saying 'no' and feeling good about protecting my time," says Rose Goldthwait, a new mom living in San Francisco. "I was able to let go of the feeling that I was obligated to be places, or be available twenty-four seven, and I let go of some work obligations. It was so foreign to me to put myself first, but I didn't want those stress chemicals in my body, and I started to see how much more resourced and whole I felt when I wasn't giving more than I had. That was some of the deepest self-care I've ever practiced."

2

Rest Well

In the early months of pregnancy, slowing down, often to a complete standstill, may be something that happens to you, rather than something you initiate. Your body is calling the shots here as it ramps up for nearly a year of hard work. Your hormones are surging and your body is holding more fluid—which can leave you anxiously awaiting your next opportunity to shut your eyes or put your feet up. "In the early days, it's about keeping the body warm and not over exerting," says Lauren. "Consume warm drinks and make room to rest." She explains that in Chinese medicine, pregnancy is considered to be a state that balances yin (mystery, stillness, and receptivity) and yang (creation, action, and output). "Pregnancy is the ultimate time in a woman's life when she is very yin, and a lot of women have not accessed that side of themselves before," she says. "It's a shock when they see that they can't do as much as they used to

> Once a pregnant person can be still, be with their breath, notice their belly, see their chest rise and fall with each inhalation and exhalation, they will come into awareness of their own voice and wisdom. We hold the key to unlock that power.
>
> —KHEFRI RILEY

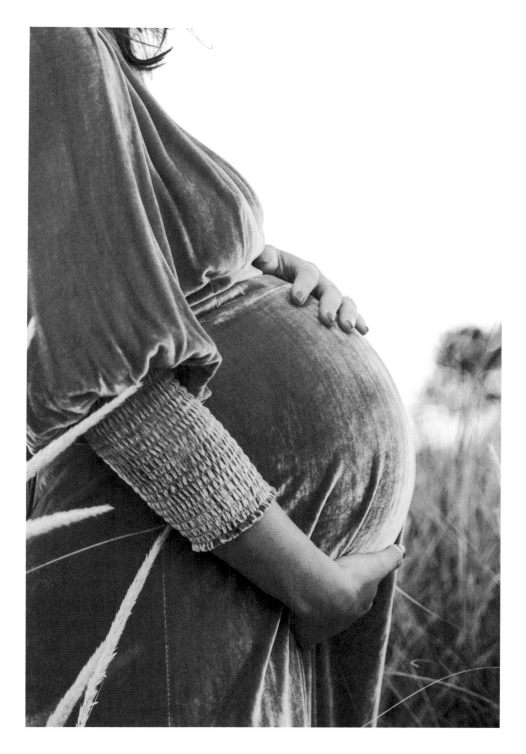

and have to get used to a new way of being. In the early weeks especially, a woman may find that she can't catch her breath as much, even walking up a slight incline, and will see that she needs to slow down because her body is changing so quickly."

A well-rested pregnancy starts with prioritizing your nightly sleep. You can sneak in pockets of rest during the day if necessary, but eight (and at times, even up to ten) hours of solid sleep will support the changes you're going through and set you up for a better birth. Traditional Ayurvedic guidelines suggest that a pregnant woman put extra emphasis on sleep during the first two and last two months of pregnancy, and aim to get to bed before 10 p.m. each night.

3

Connect with Your Baby

Your growing belly is another gateway to a regular stillness practice. It's natural to run your hands across your baby bump throughout the day, especially as it expands, but dropping into a quieter state asks you to bring intention to the experience. Spending a few minutes a day like this helps you slow down and recharge while encouraging a flourishing connection between you and your baby.

This is a time to spark the connection between you and your child. Can you tune in to their subtle messages? Some people find it easy to hear what their baby is "saying," while others still feel a bit far away from this being growing inside of them. "I offer my clients a ritual for connecting to their babies, and the feedback I receive is so touching. Even women who had issues connecting with their baby were in awe of how they could feel the baby reacting to their intention," says womb awakening mentor Ulrike Remlein. "Simply lie on your back, close your eyes, breathe gently into your belly, and place your hands on your womb where you believe your baby's head would be. Most women say they don't know where the head is, and I tell them to just pretend you know! I ask them to connect to the baby

I see that pregnant women need time to prepare to *grow into* motherhood. Yet so often they don't make time for it. My concern is that if women push it until the last minute, drop out the baby, and go into motherhood, they miss out on the sacredness of the experience.

—SIDDHI ELLINGHOVEN

with intention, offering silent or whispered words, saying, 'Beloved baby I'm here, I'm listening to you, I love you, I will show you the vast space of my womb which is your home for the next few months.' It's important to let go of expectation. The idea isn't to have something special happen; it's about having the intention of connecting to the baby. The mother can also invite the partner to connect with the baby in this way. This is a powerful practice that creates such an intimate connection to the baby and helps drop both parents into a deeply relaxed and open state."

It may seem counterintuitive to schedule time to do nothing, but factoring in regular moments of stillness and silence can become a treasured part of your pregnancy. As you dedicate time to dropping into yourself and connecting to your baby, you may find that your mind begins to settle, worrisome thoughts fading to the background as you become more comfortable in this ever-evolving experience of baby creation. Adding stillness into your daily life—remember, even five minutes of conscious breathing or meditation can make a difference in your stress and anxiety levels—will also serve as a bridge to sinking deeper into your body and all the magic it is currently conjuring up.

THE GIFT OF

HONOR

THE GIFT OF STILLNESS helps you slow down enough to see what's really going on. What you may have noticed from that quieter vantage point is that pregnancy is all about change. From one trimester to the next, or even one week to the next, you will experience a radical array of experiences in your mind, heart, and body. Whether you are moving through the first trimester or are very pregnant, there's no doubt that your body is doing things it has never done before. If this is your maiden voyage into baby making, you are experiencing the first major shift in your physiology since puberty! Your body is morphing and shifting so dramatically that it can sometimes feel strange to inhabit your own skin. Each change can take some time to adjust to—and then just when you get used to feeling a certain way, you enter a new phase and your body changes once again. It can be dizzying and disconcerting.

For starters, your period has gone on sabbatical, with an unknown date of return. Your breasts are alien creatures, tender and more bountiful than ever before. Your waistline is rapidly expanding, your ankles may be swollen, and behind the scenes, your hormones are having a raging party, taking your mood along for the ride. If you are in the early weeks, you may feel especially exhausted, dragging yourself through the day. Thankfully, things start to lift as you enter month four. The second trimester can bring a welcome spring to your step, but just as you get into the groove, the third trimester arrives, all bulky and achy, as you hobble about your day and spend hours searching for a comfortable position to sleep.

Though the changes you experience during pregnancy may seem extreme, and some of them truly are, in reality your body has always been morphing. Each phase of your menstrual cycle has been accompanied by a grab bag of emotional and physical sensations that crash in like a wave and then slip away. During each month you can experience PMS, cramps, bloating, fatigue, tender breasts, headaches, and food cravings. These sensations might take a hold of you, and then eventually release their grip. Your body will continue this hold-and-release pattern for the duration of your life—for the remainder of your pregnancy, as you give birth, in the postpartum period, throughout motherhood, and eventually menopause. Really, you are never not changing; this constant state of flux is the cyclical feminine force in action. We are designed this way, always shifting and adapting, ebbing and flowing, never static or linear. But that doesn't mean it's easy to find your footing now. The changes occurring in this phase can feel overwhelming or confusing, especially when you can no longer fit into your favorite pair of jeans or are craving nothing but fluffernutters and cold pizza.

If you had a fraught relationship with your body before you got pregnant, wishing it would look or perform differently, these nine golden months can aggravate that perspective. Pregnancy is one of the most special times of your life, but it can also be downright uncomfortable and bring up a range of feelings about what your body is doing, or not doing. You have taken on a needy tenant and there will be days when you may wonder, as you try to stuff your boobs into one of your pre-pregnancy bras or when the sight of your favorite food makes you want to barf, if your body is even yours anymore. This is natural! When you find yourself panting after walking up a tiny hill or napping under your desk at work, it is easy to feel betrayed by your body. Contrary to the images portrayed by the media, many women move through pregnancy feeling sick, achy, or just plain weird. The worst part may be that you can't control how you will feel from one day to the next—and this uncertainty can throw a monkey wrench into your already scheduled programming. If you were an earlier riser, daily runner, workaholic, overachiever, or multitasker, pregnancy can force you to scrap your plans.

The good news is you have a choice about how you respond to your physical experience. You can steel yourself against the changes happening to your body, beating yourself up about what you look like or how you feel, or you can let go and relax into the process, allowing your body to show you the way. Pregnancy can be an incredible opportunity to practice listening to the body and going with the flow. "The most important thing with pregnancy is that women trust their body and are in tune with their body," says Ulrike Remlein. "Learn to trust the signs from your body and to see it not as an enemy but as a good guide. If something is truly wrong, your body will let you know."

When you practice relaxing into your body instead of pushing against it, you will begin to move out of your head, where most of us have taken up permanent residency. Our nonstop, hyperconnected lifestyles have conditioned us to live in our minds, where stress and anxiety are born and flourish. Honoring your body through a few small gestures each day helps you step out of the mental vortex of planning, worrying, and thinking. If you have gone through life removed from the power and beauty of your body, or in a permanent tug of war with your appearance, your strength, or your energy levels, pregnancy is the ideal time to experience the opposite. "In pregnancy you are really *in* your body more than you probably ever are in your life," says new mother Jenny McNulty. There is a primal force coursing through your body during these forty weeks that can serve as a gateway into new reserves of power, potency, and joy. By honoring this phase of change for all that it is, you can move into a place of greater ease and comfort, accepting, appreciating, and even celebrating your physicality, perhaps for the first time.

Befriending Your Body

It can take some intention to tap into the positive aspects of pregnancy when it feels like you're on a roller coaster ride of emotion and sensation. You are a fierce goddess of creation one day and hobbled by back pain or nausea the next. To stay balanced through these ups and downs it helps to create conditions that encourage a happy relationship between your body and you. Consistent movement and touch practices during pregnancy will allow you to listen to your body, making it that much easier to advocate for yourself during the heightened experience of birth. You will be able to declare, "This feels good right now," or "I want to move in this way," or "Please don't touch me like that." Of course, every ounce of love you give your body influences your baby's experience too. Just imagine if, as the ancient ways shared, everything you taste, see, touch, and feel is experienced by your baby. Wouldn't you want to make the time to tend to yourself, to tap into the sense of reverence and awe that comes when you honor your body? You get back twice what you put in—good feelings for you, and for your little one too.

During pregnancy, you are fielding the ideas and opinions of so many people—care providers, friends, family, and your partner. You're poring through books, websites, and YouTube videos about how to have a healthy pregnancy and an easeful birth. You may be poked and prodded, assessed, and stared at. But just as you can decide to find moments of stillness when the world is rushing all around you, choosing to honor your body through movement or touch helps you remember that regardless of what anyone says, whether they have a degree on the wall or not, this is your body and your experience. Furthermore, tending to your body deliberately and kindly can help reconnect you to something you might not always hear speaking to you: your instinct. When we are in touch with this nonintellectual awareness, we tend to feel safer in our own skin and more confident in the choices we make. "At any time in your life, it's great to connect with your body so you can hear your intuition, but in navigating pregnancy, it's actually essential to have ways to check in with yourself and listen," says Rochelle Schieck. "There are a million different decisions and opinions to sift through; to go through that process without having a strong sense of your own self makes it beyond challenging." Haize Hawke, who has supported many birthing people to deliver their babies, encourages deep connection to the body throughout pregnancy, in order to be ready for the final stages. "One of the many challenges in labor and delivery is to stay out of the *thinking* body and drop into the *feeling* body. Walking the birthing labyrinth is all about listening to the body, honoring the intuition, and trusting the process. I always say, 'Don't think your way through, *feel* your way through.'" She and other wise ones describe how mothers who activate this body sense early on in their pregnancies are fortified with a profound level of self-belief by the time baby is ready to come—I am exquisitely designed to do this; I have everything I need to do it.

So how *do* you listen to your body and let it speak a bit louder than your mind, you might ask? Add small doses of three simple things to your days, as best you can: Movement, Touch, and Beauty.

> I found that there was a missed opportunity to celebrate all that your body can do during pregnancy. I wanted to reframe the conversation from pregnancy being a prognosis to it being a rite of passage, a continuation of the lineage of humanity, or a spiritual state—not a medical condition that you have to manage.
>
> —ROCHELLE SCHIECK, *founder of Qoya*

Movement

At this point in your life, you've likely tuned into just how supportive regular movement can be for a positive state of body and mind. It's just as much so during pregnancy. Movement not only strengthens your muscles and improves your cardiovascular health, it releases chemicals that help you feel happier, more hopeful, and even more connected to others. And on a subtler level, it wakes up your ability to respond to your body—to truly be with it and connect. "Many of us ignore our body's messaging, by doing habitual things like turning to coffee when we're tired instead of resting or drinking more water," says Rochelle Schieck, who developed

Without movement, you would be missing out on an opportunity to deeply connect with yourself. A regular movement practice gives you a deeper understanding of yourself so you are better equipped to navigate all of the different decisions and opinions coming your way.

—ROCHELLE SCHIECK

her women's movement modality, Qoya (a fusion of yoga, creative dance expression, and ritual), to help women remember that their essence is wild, wise, and free and to trust in the truths they hold inside their bodies. She finds that when women allow themselves to drop into movement, they start to feel with their senses those deeper things that their minds were too busy to detect, like what they need to experience more of to feel well, or what they need to let go of, or what they are longing for in order to feel nurtured and held. This knowing can serve as an inner compass during birth as you move through the various stages of labor; you will be more equipped to ask for the support you need in each moment.

Most traditions of pregnancy care advocate for a gentle approach to movement in the first trimester. It may feel outdated to proceed with caution in the early weeks of pregnancy, but rather than feeling constricted or limited, can you see this early phase of pregnancy as a tender moment deserving of awareness and discernment? "CrossFit workouts and other strenuous exercises can put a lot of strain on the pelvic floor; it's good to leave that alone in the early stages of pregnancy and wait," cautions Lauren Curtain. "Likewise, the marathon runner will need to slow it down. I suggest going for restorative movement like walking, gentle yoga, gentle Pilates, and not pushing too hard." There's a good chance you will feel invincible later in pregnancy, and certainly with the right coaching from those well versed in pregnancy physiology, you may feel great lifting weights too, a little further down the line. But allow yourself to experiment with softer ways of moving. Rather than feeling like you are losing out on exercise, can you give yourself permission to abandon the need to keep up with your old self?

Walking

Sometimes the simplest forms of exercise are the most profound. Whether you were a triathlete before pregnancy or rarely put on your sneakers, walking is the physical outlet most often recommended by midwives. "At our practice, we are major proponents of walking," says Davi Khalsa. "I used to recommend that women walk five miles a day. Now I say, anything you can do is fantastic." Walking regularly during pregnancy can lower the risk of developing gestational diabetes, slow weight gain (which helps avoid premature birth), bring relief from back pain, help you sleep better, and relieve constipation. It's possible to simply put one foot in front of the other and receive the immense benefits of walking, but when you bring some mindfulness to how your body is moving through space, you elevate the experience.

As you walk, bring your attention to your feet as they touch the ground. Can you feel the four corners of each foot—the ball of the foot under the big and pinkie toes, and the left and right sides of the heel? Notice the muscles in your legs as they activate to carry your forward. What happens when you go up or down a hill? There are a variety of sensations moving through your body as you walk. Some may be positive, warming, and energizing, while others may be uncomfortable with tension, tightness, or pain. It's all part of the experience! Whether walking is easy and enlivening or slightly challenging (always avoid walking if you're in pain, and talk to your care provider if you have any concerns), whether you're hiking in the forest or strolling around your neighborhood, use each walk as an opportunity to appreciate the vitality and power of your body—you're growing a human being and moving through space. You're pretty much a miracle in motion!

Yoga

You will be hard pressed to find a care provider who doesn't applaud the benefits of yoga during pregnancy. Whether you were an advanced yogi pre-pregnancy, sweating it out in Ashtanga classes, or you're brand-new to the ancient practice, the gentle and strengthening postures of prenatal yoga (yoga that's been modified to support the specific needs of a pregnant woman) can keep you strong and healthy during these forty weeks and prepare you for the specific demands of birth. Yoga is not your average exercise. The stretching and strengthening movements are paired with conscious breathing to give you more bang for your buck—physical well-being plus mental and emotional calming: fit and peaceful. Nods to the physical discipline of hatha yoga can be found throughout Ayurvedic texts, praising it for its nurturing qualities and for the way it uses the breath to help the practitioner ride waves of effort and release. In yoga, you may be softening into a deep stretch

I tell women, as you go through your yoga asanas, your baby is doing theirs! They go through all their positions, their asanas, their mudras, I think they do it all! I think babies are so in tune with the infinite; they *are* infinity.

—DAVI KHALSA

or activating the muscles in an energized pose. In working this way, you become intimately familiar with surrender and power and learn how to relate to your body with compassion and respect.

Yoga is a different way into physical self-care; regardless of how hard you're working on your mat, it will never require the exertion of a spin class or a five-mile run. You may break a sweat while moving through yoga asanas (postures), but you won't be pushing yourself into true discomfort (or at least you shouldn't be). Your muscles will become strong and toned—and practicing yoga throughout pregnancy offers the added benefit of training your body to access tranquility. "In my yoga classes and my prenatal training, the primary focus is regulation of the nervous system," says Siddhi Ellinghoven. "We calm the mother's nervous system and calm the baby's nervous system. I bring them into expansion and contraction, so it becomes a pattern. The movements become a metaphor for the day of labor. By the time labor arrives they know how to ride the waves of the breath, using it to invite the sensation in, rather than resisting it—when you allow the sensation, there can be less discomfort." Make it to your mat regularly during pregnancy and you'll slide into birth strong, calm, and prepared to handle anything that comes your way.

Stay Open with Cat-Cow

If you do one yoga pose during your pregnancy, make it cat-cow. The simple pose offers a wealth of benefits and feels so good at every stage of pregnancy. A few rounds of cat-cow each day for thirty seconds to a minute can help to relieve back pain and keep length and mobility in the spine.

Come to all fours, with your hands below the shoulders, and knees aligned with the hips. As you inhale, curl the tailbone and lift the heart and head up. If you feel tension in the belly, keep your gaze toward the floor.

As you exhale, curl the tailbone in (arching your back like a cat), bringing the chin to the chest and feeling the palms root into the floor. This should give you a gentle spinal stretch. Repeat four to six times, with long, slow inhales and exhales.

Ditch Gravity. Go Swimming.

As your body morphs to accommodate your growing baby, getting out of a chair or walking up a hill can become surprising feats of athleticism. Your body may feel heavier than ever before and you can find yourself counting down the minutes until you can rest your swollen feet. If everything feels like it's tugging you down, you may want to skip movement practices that keep you tethered to the ground and try something deliciously weightless. Swimming is a wonderful way to get moving during pregnancy without the hassle of gravity. Enter a body of water and suddenly you're not so heavy anymore; plus, suspending yourself in water mimics your baby's experience in the womb, dropping you and your little one into an intimately shared experience. You can swim gentle laps or use a float or the side of the wall (if you're in a pool) to kick your legs. Salty ocean water is always healing, but your local pool will also do the trick.

Dance

There is no better time than pregnancy to dance like nobody's watching. Shaking your booty is a joyful way to move energy, burn some calories, and get you out of your head and into your body. Anyone can dance—even if you have two left feet! When guiding women through Qoya, Rochelle Schieck encourages them to focus on what feels good. The recipe? Skip the complex choreography, pump up the jams, and simply move. You don't need to be a savvy DJ to get the beats pumpin'. Rochelle uses the randomness of the shuffle feature—she calls this the "Oracle Shuffle"—to decide how she'll move. Simply put on a playlist, press "shuffle," and give it over to a higher power to organize how it comes out. Whatever song comes up, dance to that and notice how it makes you feel, really landing in the moment. You can do this for just three to five minutes whenever you're feeling the need to move. "There's no way you can do it wrong," reminds Rochelle. "Ask yourself, 'how can I move in a way that helps me feel the most like myself?' And then trust that physical sensation of truth in your body; it's a resonance that can be felt. This is the shift from the mind to the body—instead of thinking your way through, you're feeling. Tapping into that felt sense is an essential part of preparing for birth."

When it comes to getting your boogie on, it's not about mastering the tango or channeling Beyoncé. The goal here is to simply move some stagnant energy and get your heart rate up a bit, always with the awareness that your baby is settling in for the coming months. Dancing also happens to be an efficient way to get your happy juices pumping, busting right through melancholy or lethargy. Be sure to give the hips some special attention, circling them and swaying back and forth—this helps open the pelvis, preparing the way for giving birth. If you're worried about impact, keep your feet on the floor. You don't need to leave the ground to benefit from dancing. Rock your hips, stick out your rear end, shrug your shoulders, and shake out your arms, wrists, and hands. Pay close attention to the movements that feel good to you (and do more of them!) and notice what doesn't feel good. Dancing should be a joyful, playful expression. If it hurts, stop and try something else. All the micro adjustments you make as you dance are a pure practice of listening in and responding—fortifying your trust in yourself like nothing else.

Make a commitment to have a mini dance party a couple times a week. Blast your favorite tunes and dance with your child, your partner, your pet, or yourself. You can try out a few belly dancing videos on YouTube or keep it freeform—just see if you can keep moving from the start to the end of a song. Bounce, shake, and shimmy, and when the song is over, stand perfectly still and notice how you feel.

Finding Peace When It's Hard

Pregnancy can bring up discomforts that, out of caution for baby's health, you might not be able to numb away with a pill. If you have a headache, a cold, a cramped lower back, sciatica, indigestion, another physical challenge, or are managing a condition you had before you were pregnant, the undeniable truth is that you're going to face hard days that you just can't escape from. This is a huge practice of surrender and acceptance. Like the sensations you'll experience in labor, pain and discomfort during pregnancy ask you to ride the waves of what you're feeling, and instead of contracting around what hurts, to relax, soften, and release. "I have a pinched nerve in my back and normally I would take a painkiller for it, but I didn't want to do anything that could possibly harm the baby," says new mom Rose Goldthwait. "So it was more about saying, this hurts, and it sucks right now. This is what it is. It's about remembering that it is a season—it's going to pass."

Touch

"Whatever form it takes—cuddles, kisses, stroking, lovemaking—touch is a huge component of well-being for the mother-to-be," says Damian Hagglund, Ayurvedic marma therapy practitioner. "Touch is as important as food and hydration." If you are in a partnership, pregnancy is an ideal time to connect physically. It can be as simple as stroking your back, lightly scratching your scalp, or even a nurturing foot rub, which is especially good for grounding and relaxing any anxiety that results from naturally elevated vata dosha. (Just be sure not to apply pressure around the ankles, due to pressure points there that can stimulate contractions.) Aim for light caresses rather than vigorous Swedish rubdowns (again, to avoid stimulating any pressure points that can induce labor)—save the full-body massages for a professional prenatal massage therapist.

Your main squeeze doesn't have to have bodyworker skills to support you in this way. The simple act of offering you purposeful touch is one filled with love. Your job— harder than it sounds, sometimes—is to practice letting go of the need to be productive, busy, or useful, and to really receive these gestures of care.

> There are so many ways to feel yourself from the inside. For some, it's meditation; for some, it's shaking and dancing. All are ways to come back to yourself.
>
> —SIDDHI ELLINGHOVEN

I Like It Like That

Rochelle Schieck suggests using touch not simply to relax your body, but also to invigorate your voice. "I recommend a simple massage ritual where the partner offers the pregnant woman a massage and she practices expressing exactly how she feels in the moment, clearly requesting, 'Can you do it a little harder?' or 'Can you do it a little softer?' The person offering the massage simply hears her requests and honors them without taking anything personally. This is an exercise to get the pregnant woman comfortable with stating her needs, where in the past perhaps she would have said, 'Oh, it's fine,' when she was really longing for something else. It's a great practice to prepare for birth, where it will be essential to express your preferences for touch and support to your partner, and for them to respond with neutrality, as they arise and change."

GIVE YOURSELF THE GIFT OF ABHYANGA

Self-massage is a beautiful way to honor your changing body throughout your pregnancy. Abhyanga (Sanskrit for "oil massage") is the simple, timeless Ayurvedic practice of massaging warm oil into the body from head to toe. Applying oil to the body is calming, grounding, and relaxing—an instant stress reliever. This ritual is a way of offering love to yourself and your baby while also helping decrease stretch marks, maintain the skin's elasticity, and temper itching that can occur as your belly stretches to accommodate your little one. And it's easy! Warm some unrefined, organic sesame oil or another carrier oil of choice (listed on page 250) by setting a jar of it in hot water until warm. Apply using an open palm—long strokes on your long bones and circular strokes on the joints. Massage all of you, gently applying the oil to your belly. Notice which areas of your body are more tense than others. Do you feel heightened sensitivity around your navel? Are your breasts tender to the touch? Follow the massage with a warm bath or shower to support circulation. You can amp up the appreciation for all that your body is doing by softly saying "thank you" as you run your hands over each part of your body. Thank you, feet, for carrying me through each day. Thank you, hands, for creating and working. Thank you, womb, for growing my baby. It may feel silly at first, but this clear expression of gratitude is like making a deposit in your self-love bank account. Do it enough times and your funds will be overflowing; you will truly believe in your body's ability to carry, birth, and raise this child with ease and grace.

Receiving touch from another person can feel really good, but you don't have to rely on anyone else to honor yourself in this way. You can easily give yourself the gift of touch by finding a few minutes, ideally each day, but anytime you can, to connect to your own body with devotion and intention. Give yourself a massage with an organic massage oil infused with a few drops of essential oil. Use the mix-and-match guidelines for massage oil on page 250, experimenting with different scents. The simple commitment to giving yourself purposeful touch creates an instant atmosphere of self-love and appreciation for the changing landscape of your body. "Pregnancy is the ultimate expression of the female form. With big, juicy boobs and a growing tummy, it's all about femininity," says Lauren Curtain. "If a woman is used to being small or less curvy, this change can be confronting. For some, having boobs that are bigger than ever is a clear yes, but others feel self-conscious about taking up more room. I remind women that you can expand—this is a time of expansion and growth!—and it's not going to last forever. I love seeing a woman embrace how her body is changing." Whether you indulge in a head-to-toe Abhyanga massage (see opposite), simply rub the kinks out of your hands and feet (if you can still touch them!), or do the Breast Care ritual (page 250), taking the time to nurture and appreciate yourself drops you and baby into a blissful state.

If massage isn't your thing, you can boost your oxytocin and honor your body by getting snuggly. Spoon with your partner (your growing belly may require that you be the little spoon), have a solo retreat under some warm blankets (if you're feeling anxious or worried, choose covers with some weight, as the pressure has been found to soothe the nervous system), or cozy up to your pet. Finding time to step away from the outside world into a warm and nurturing space is a way of telling your body that you appreciate all that it's doing and want to reward it with a much needed respite.

What's on Your Skin?

You have the opportunity during every moment of pregnancy to create an optimal sensory experience for your body. Everything that you put on, and in, your body offers you the chance to elevate your experience. There's a good chance that you have already been adjusting your personal care routine to include only products made from natural, plant-derived ingredients. If you're new to the rapidly growing world of clean beauty, check out the Environmental Working Group (ewg.org) to learn more about the sea of unregulated chemicals that are found in the products we use every day, from deodorant to shampoo and makeup. Thankfully, there are many effective (and luxurious) safe personal care products on the market today—and since everything you place on your skin is absorbed into your bloodstream, pregnancy is an ideal time to do an inventory of the products taking residency in your bathroom and to clean house where necessary.

The sense of honoring your body during pregnancy extends to the clothes you wear as well. What feels good on your skin? Are there certain textures and colors that help you feel relaxed and free? If you are expecting during the summer or live in a warm climate, look for clothing that has a light, breezy feel to it—if you've always leaned toward body-hugging clothing, this is a good time to try something different—muumuu, anyone? If it's chilly, find cozy items that help you feel warm and cared for: a colorful scarf or a favorite knit hat. Choosing natural fibers (cotton, silk, linen, wool, etc.) is always a good bet as synthetics don't allow the skin to breathe and can irritate sensitive skin.

Beauty

Honoring yourself during pregnancy consistently comes back to beauty. How deeply can you appreciate the beauty of your strong and capable body? Do you notice, and absorb, the small moments of beauty that you encounter each day? This is a lot easier to do once you have made it through the awkwardness and uncertainty of the first trimester. The first months of pregnancy can be filled with nausea, fatigue, and anxiety, but in the second trimester many women start to feel vibrant and juicy, like a ripe peach.

This is a great time to extend the self-love you stoked with dancing, yoga, or massage and consciously slather yourself with some appreciation for just how marvelous you are. Hire a professional photographer to document you at this special stage of life, or take some artsy selfies! Even if you go on to have many more babies, you'll never look exactly like this again. "I would encourage every pregnant woman to hire someone to take really beautiful portraits," says our photographer Jenny McNulty. "You can look back and say, 'That was me, that was my body.' It's a worthwhile investment, even if you don't feel confident and beautiful. Do it anyway, so you can see how everyone else is seeing you. Having that record is really important."

Create a Daily Beauty Practice

Integrating more beauty into your life can be as easy as asking yourself, "What beauty is around me today?" Not sure? Start by looking up. What color is the sky? Can you feel the sun's rays warming the top of your head and cheeks? Are there any trees or flowers nearby? Create a daily beauty practice by going on a nature walk or making a cup of tea and sitting in a cozy spot, gazing upon a favorite plant or art print. If you don't have a beautiful nook in which to perch, this is the time to make one. Create a beautiful nest now and it will be your special beauty spot during pregnancy—and during the first forty days while you're busy feeding and soothing your baby. Build a space with inspiring art and objects, cozy throw pillows and blankets, and plants. Even paint a wall in a color you love. (Choose no-VOC paint if possible.) You don't need a lot of space; a corner of your bedroom or a slice of the living room will suffice. This will be your place to recharge, retreat, and fill your mind and heart with beauty.

In Bali, Ibu Robin Lim encourages each of the mothers receiving care at her center, Bumi Sehat, to recognize how magnificent they are, specifically noticing their unique beauty, a beauty that is reflected in the natural environment that surrounds them. ("Bumi" means "earth mother" and "sehat" means "healthy.") "As women, loving ourselves and appreciating our own beauty really contributes to our happiness," she says. Robin applies this self-love to herself as well. "I like to start and end my day with a little prayer of appreciation for all the blessings in my life: my family, my home, my village, the sun above and the rain that makes our food grow, the air we breathe, my garden, and my healthy beautiful body." The midwives at Bumi Sehat also carry an appreciation of beauty into their daily interactions with birthing mothers. One of the midwives on the team has been practicing midwifery for forty-two years and makes a little extra effort to show up for her mothers. "She puts on makeup every day before coming to work—I never do that!" laughs Robin. "When I asked her about it, she told me, 'I put on my

WHEN THE BEAUTY IS HARD TO FIND

It's easy to write about magic and beauty, but we do so understanding that there will be some moments during pregnancy when the rainbows and sunshine are especially elusive. You are a human being having a very human experience. Pregnant or not, there will be times when you feel light, open, and hopeful, and others where you feel heavy, dark, or uncertain. Though it's easier to feel happy, we are designed to experience a full range of emotions, and that includes the tougher ones. The challenge is to allow the entire spectrum of emotions to come up without rejecting them, distracting yourself away from them, or judging them. When you give a feeling space to exist without attaching a bigger story to it, that feeling will move through you and another one will be right behind it—just as clouds move across the sky. You are not your anxiety or your melancholy; you are so much bigger than any one feeling you experience. You are the sky.

Your main work as a becoming mother is to raise your frequency. Be aware of what serves you—and what takes away from you.

-SIDDHI ELLINGHOVEN

lipstick because I want my face to say "I love you" to the woman in labor or having her checkup; I do it for my women, so they feel the love.'"

What would it be like if every step you took during pregnancy was on a bed of rose petals? If the air around you was scented with the fragrance of jasmine and wisteria, and your eyes were filled with rolling green vistas and bright blue skies? The ancient ones wanted that much beauty to fill the senses of the pregnant person, but you don't need to live in a magical fairyland to get a daily dose of beauty. Whether you're tethered to your computer, working intensely throughout your pregnancy, navigating the same commute through an urban landscape, or juggling family responsibilities with your partner and other child(ren), with a bit of conscious intention, you can infuse traces of beauty into the most mundane of days. The quickest, and cheapest, route to filling yourself with beauty is to recognize the bounty of the natural world. Whether you live in a city, the suburbs, or deep in the country, nature is always there for you. Leaning into the stillness practices you learned in Treasure One, take some time to downshift and notice what's around you, or above you. See the trees, the flowers, the sunset. Mother Nature is abundant and it costs nothing to take in her bounty. Don't miss out on this direct route to folding more beauty into your life.

> Each time you catch your own image in the mirror, try to say this simple blessing to yourself: "You are so beautiful, I love you."
>
> —ROBIN LIM

Honoring your body for its wisdom, magnificence, and infinite capacity to grow and birth your baby is a stepping stone along the way to deeply trusting yourself. And it doesn't have to be hard! Simple movement, touch, and beauty practices can help you tune into what works—and doesn't work—for you. This is a profoundly personal kind of knowing that will support you throughout your parenting journey.

THE GIFT OF

TRUST

FTER SPENDING TIME with Treasure Two, you hopefully discovered that getting to know and appreciate your body is a worthy investment. Through each downward dog or kitchen dance party, in every oil massage or foot rub, you stepped deeper through the doorway of feeling more at home in your skin. Perhaps a sense of safety starts to grow, or relaxation, or even empowerment as you regularly step out of the busy terrain of the mind.

Settled into your physical vessel, you will be better prepared to field the many decisions surrounding pregnancy, birth, and early motherhood that seem to increase in velocity and importance as you get closer to the big day. You may be weighing major issues, like the pros and cons of a home birth, finding a doula who truly feels like a fit, or even arguing with your partner over circumcision. And pushed up right next to those significant decisions are the smaller moment-to-moment questions, like whether it's OK to have that glass of wine or another piece of pie, or to take on that extra project at work.

You may make the decision to undergo an intervention suggested by your care provider or to decline a social invite that would likely leave you more fatigued than inspired. Whatever you choose is the right choice! You are the captain of this ship—it is your body, and your baby, and you get to decide what feels right. But to get to that confident place of knowing, you first have to be able to trust yourself to understand what works for you and what doesn't. Before becoming pregnant, you may not have had to consider your level of self-trust. When faced with a fork in the road, you may have explored the various sides of each decision and marched forth without deeply contemplating, Do I trust myself to know what's best for me? Maybe you even sought answers outside of yourself, looking to others to tell you what to do. You're not alone. "Many women come to the pregnancy and birth experience with an unconscious conditioning that their bodies are not trustworthy," says Rochelle Schieck. "Pregnancy then offers an incredible opportunity for each person to ask themselves, 'How can I trust myself and my body more through this experience?'"

You can go through pregnancy as you've always done, doing your best to think your way through each choice you face, or handing the decision-making over to somebody outside of yourself—a caregiver, your partner, a parent, or a friend. Or you can make a commitment to use this pivotal moment in your life, on the threshold of becoming a Mother, or Mother Again, to take full responsibility for each decision you make, sourcing guidance not only from your thinking mind or anybody on the outside, but also from a deep well of self-trust that lives within you. Our wise ones tell us, and we've seen firsthand in our own mothering journeys, that pregnancy comes most alive with meaning when you step into the driver's seat of your experience, owning each step you choose to take along the way. Accessing this current of trust can take some practice, but as with the first two treasures, the greatest motivation to experiment with these new ways of being is right inside you—your baby and his or her well-being.

It can be easy to get swept away by the sheer adorableness of a pair of tiny booties, daydreaming about holding your little one in your arms. There is a sweetness and joy to the pregnancy experience, of course, and you deserve to enjoy all of it, yet there's no denying that the stakes are high here. You are at the epicenter of one of the most significant moments of your life: growing a human being inside of your body, delivering that being into the world, and then tending to it for eighteen years, if not for life. If you are not grounded in a strong, confident place of self-trust throughout your pregnancy, into your birth experience, and during motherhood, it will be too easy to get tugged along by a medical system that may not understand, or want to understand, what really feels right for you, or to cave into fears, uncertainty, or shame that you're not doing it right. Tapping into your inner trust can serve as an anchor point that will give you the strength to ride the waves of this experience, and to make decisions that sometimes feel like life or death.

Becoming attuned to your inner guidance system—the place that tells you that you need to get in or out of the birthing tub during labor, or that you don't need to take that glucose test, or that you need more alone time, or more together time—is actually not such a big leap from where you are right now. Being in an active state of baby creation automatically sets you up for greater empathy and compassion. You may be getting weepy at commercials or find yourself filled with gushing appreciation when a friend gives you her

> When we assert intuition, we are therefore like the starry night: We gaze at the world through a thousand eyes.
>
> —CLARISSA PINKOLA ESTÉS

favorite pair of pregnancy pants or your coworker texts you a sweet meme about motherhood. You may also be worrying more about the future. All of this is normal and healthy, and a signpost of the seismic shift that is happening inside you. You are becoming more open and sensitive. This new state can feel empowering, but it can also be unsettling if you have not touched on this side of yourself before. The windfall of emotions and the red, or green, flags now waving from your inner place of knowing, your seat of self-trust and intuition, can be overwhelming. Rochelle warns pregnant women to "get ready to explode in every direction—in the joy direction, in the grief direction, in the trust direction . . . and in the fear direction."

BREATHE OUT THE HARD STUFF

Lori Bregman is a Los Angeles–based doula, a good friend of MotherBees, and author of *The Mindful Mom-to-Be*. This is her go-to when pregnancy jitters hit.

- Find a comfortable position, seated or lying down with pillows under your head and knees.

- Inhale slowly through your nose for the count of four, hold for two, exhale out through the mouth for the count of five or more.

- Now breathe a feeling of peace deep into your belly and exhale any stress out through your mouth.

- Inhale faith; exhale doubt.

- Inhale love; exhale fear.

- Inhale health and vitality; exhale sickness or disease.

- Inhale tranquility; exhale tension.

- Inhale happiness and joy; exhale sadness or disappointment.

- Inhale something you long for; exhale any blocks to having it.

- Inhale something you want to increase (joy, laugher, connection, etc.); exhale something you'd like to decrease (worry, fear, anxiety, sadness, etc.).

- Inhale the present moment; exhale the past. (It's over.)

- Inhale the present moment; exhale the future (It hasn't happened yet.)

- Inhale the present moment; exhale the present moment . . . and be here now.

This explosion of feeling is a key aspect of pregnancy, and if you nurture this part of yourself, rather than shutting it down or judging it, it will help ignite your intuition superpower. In fact, your increased sensitivity goes hand in hand with building trust in yourself, one supporting the other, the trust helping you remain grounded as swirls of vulnerability and fear attempt to yank you out of what you know to be true. Your trust in yourself is like the roots of an old oak tree, digging deep into the earth to stabilize you as you stretch taller into new chapters of yourself and navigate any challenging situations that arise. Without this stability, you can be pulled into the thoughts and opinions of others—which tend to run plentiful around pregnant and birthing women and new mothers. It's important to establish the roots of self-trust in pregnancy, so you are able to access it if you have to make a split-second decision while giving birth. Meditation teacher and mother Yashoda Devi Ma reminds her students that this is the time to stand strong in your decisions, whether that's with care providers or your partner or other family members. "If you don't own your path, they will guide you through fear," she says. "It really takes a lot of courage to stand up and say, 'This is the path that I'm taking, and you guys need to go with it or keep your mouth shut—I'm so certain of what I want in this instance, I actually don't want to hear what you have to say.'"

> The less you think, examine, study, and read, the more time you have to be in your intuition. My wife and I would read little bits of information about pregnancy, then go for a walk. We would walk multiple times a day. You contemplate, you walk, you talk. You want to digest the info so you can process it and see how you would act upon it or not, asking yourselves, "Do we even agree with this?"
>
> —DAMIAN HAGGLUND

In some ways, learning to hear the whispers of your intuition, which starts by practicing stillness and then honoring the wisdom of your body, is easier today than it has ever been—if only because you have more opportunities to feel into what lands as "true" for you. Thanks to social media, moms-to-be have instant access to people who are stepping into their own power during pregnancy and birth, with striking images of fierce birthing mamas and their deeply authentic shares. Yet, simultaneously, the internet asks birthing people to weed through more information and manage greater isolation than they've ever faced before.

Though you may want to stand up strong and own every decision that is true for you, without keen awareness, anxiety and doubt can begin to chip away at your resolve—it can be challenging to sense what feels really right when so much is coming at you.

It's important to remember that self-trust is a process of becoming more of who you really are. It can take time, and you will never run out of opportunities to practice, starting from where you are in this exact moment in time, through birth, and into a lifetime of mothering. "In becoming a mother, you are signing up for the spiritual teaching of your life," says Michelle Price, a mother of two in California. "Really, you are birthing your spiritual teacher, and this thing is going to teach you more about what you're made of than anything else. It's like a marathon that lasts your whole life, where you're always in a process of shedding your skin, trying to figure out 'Who am I?' There were moments when I definitely felt like a stranger to myself."

Get to Know Your Fear

Pregnancy is a time to work through any fears that may be coming up around your growing baby's safety, the birth process, and becoming a mother. We're not talking about conquering or eliminating your fears completely, because that's just not possible. It's more about bringing them to the surface so they're not unconsciously controlling your experience. When fears are pushed aside or covered up, they remain unresolved and can get between you and your intuition. Self-trust is cultivated when every part of you, even the aspects that you are ashamed about or dislike, are given space at the table.

We'd rather go to a psychic or astrologer than go within and hear the answer.

—DAVI KHALSA

Fear can also be stoked by taking in too much information. You may find your mind buzzing after a few hours reading articles online, scrolling Instagram feeds about pregnancy and birth, and devouring yet another book about fetal development. If you're already feeling unsure about what decision to make, ingesting too much information can begin to consume you, leaving you confused and disoriented. "A woman will oftentimes say, 'I don't know how I feel,' and I always love to reassure her: *You do*. I say, 'You're feeling

PRACTICING FEARLESSNESS

Yashoda Devi Ma teaches how the conscious use of sound and vibration can help shift our thinking, remove our stuck emotions, and release stress from the body. Here, she shares sound in the form of a mantra ("man" = "mind"; "tra" = "transport"), a sacred vibration that can help you enter a deep state of meditation. When fear rises, she suggests using the bija mantra LAM (pronounced "lahm"), because its vibration is connected to the root chakra, which is said to store our fears. Practiced regularly, this mantra can help you become fearless.

- Sit in a comfortable upright position with your spine tall. Close your eyes and soften the area around your heart.

- Relax your body and release your mind of control and judgment. (When we meditate, all thoughts and emotions are accepted; everything is good and nothing is bad.)

- Breathe in through the nose and out through the mouth, allowing the inhalations and exhalations to be long, smooth, and full.

- Exhale all tension, stress, anxiety, and fear. Continue breathing like this for three minutes, ending with an exhalation out the mouth.

- Keep the eyes closed and introduce the bija mantra: "LAM" ("lahm").

- Start by saying the mantra out loud so the body and baby can feel the vibration of the sound as it ripples through the water of the body.

- Inhale through the nose and exhale out the mouth while saying the mantra "LAM." Inhale and exhale the mantra.

- Repeat for four minutes, whispering the mantra for the last minute.

- Repeat the mantra silently for three minutes or up to ten minutes. Slowly open eyes.

a lot of different feelings, so let's take a few breaths and slow down, because you *do* know,'" explains Davi Khalsa, who regularly brings yogic practices and mindfulness into her midwifery care. "Mostly she's overwhelmed because she has taken in too much information. The more books a woman reads, the further she disconnects from her own feelings." She advises her clients to briefly center themselves with a one-minute meditation or chant when confusion hits. "I'll say, 'Do you feel that feeling?' They say 'yes,' and I'll say, 'That is you connecting with you. You really know how you feel, but you get overwhelmed with so much information and other people telling you how you should be acting, feeling, and looking.' This helps her drop into the experience of feeling herself!"

Permission to Pause

In my own postpartum experience, I was reading all the books on how to be the best mom and how to raise the healthiest kid, and one day I swear I opened up the window and threw all the books outside because they were preventing me from getting in touch with my feelings. I didn't trust myself, and that's what I think a lot of women come face-to-face with along the mothering journey. Sometimes we need more help, it's true, but it starts by connecting with the truth within, by slowing down inside of ourselves so that we can actually feel what we are feeling, and connect with our own truth. —Davi Khalsa

Wait! Before you toss all of your books—and iPhone—out the window, please know that information is absolutely invited to this party. The key is finding that sweet spot between knowledge and wisdom—between the head (where rational thinking resides) and the heart (where intuition lives). Having a clear understanding of pregnancy and birth, including your options and potential risks and challenges, will empower you to be able to listen to your intuition, and to know what's really best for you and your baby. Once you are armed with information, you will be better equipped to recognize fear when it comes up in you.

Let's be real: Researching is an inevitable part of the modern woman's pregnancy journey. With twenty-four seven access to an entire universe of content, often just a few clicks away on your phone, it can be challenging to resist the siren call of information. If you're feeling research fatigue, turn your sights to a more participatory form of information gathering. A childbirth preparation class can be an excellent way to understand how birth works without cramming your brain full of the written word. Attending a class gets you out of the house, can be a bonding experience with your partner (and will give them a chance to be part of the experience), and is a way to be an active participant in this experience. "When the subject of birth comes up, a lot of women say, 'I don't even want to think about it'; they push it out of their mind," says Lauren Curtain. "I believe you need to be as invested in your birth as you would when moving into a new house. You don't just turn up and hope for the best! You need to understand the lingo, to be familiar with the terminology. If you default to just doing what your OB says, you may end up with unnecessary intervention. It's your body, your baby, and your birth—and your decisions determine how it will go."

> In pregnancy, you need to be more in your intuition than ever, but I am not sure that comes easily because we are taught from an early age that pregnancy is a time to rely on others, that doctors will tell you what's going on and what to do or not to do. I found that individual self-knowing is the hardest component to learn; you can't really be taught how to do it.
>
> —JENNY MCNULTY, *new mother*

Who's Your Person?

When feelings of doubt, shame, or embarrassment come up, it can be tempting to stay silent, internalizing these hard emotions. The antidote is to find at least one safe space to voice your feelings. This could be with a trusted friend or family member—someone who understands the power of listening without advising—a therapist, clergy member, or a midwife, doula, your OB, or another non-judgmental care provider. It's time to ask: Who's my person?

A Closer Look at Intuition

Trusting yourself exists in direct relation to how clearly you can connect to your intuition—but what is intuition exactly? "I always describe it as a nonlinear felt sense," says Rochelle Schieck. "The mind is always going to grab onto things that are literal and linear—things that make logical sense. Intuition is the opposite, the nonlinear felt sense. It's like when you're looking at art. There's not a right or wrong way to experience it—you like it or you don't like it, that's it. That's what intuition is; you feel drawn toward something or you don't. This doesn't mean that you're actively looking for an answer; it's more about tracking resonance, a word that I often use in place of intuition. Resonance is when something has a feeling-based association, as if your body is a tuning fork and you are attuning to something."

Intuition or resonance is like our sixth sense, an invisible guidance system that alerts us to whether or not something feels right (i.e., safe) for us. Intuition is a different kind of knowing than rational thinking or reasoning. We are all born with this primal ability to instinctively know if we are heading in the right direction; it's the gut feeling we get when something is off—or on. But as we move deeper into society, with its barrage of distraction and stimulation, we can also move farther away from this knowing place within us. We can start to doubt that voice inside us—and when we discount it long enough, it can eventually go dormant. Thankfully, it's never too late to reintroduce yourself to your intuition, and there's no better time to practice than the forty-ish weeks of pregnancy. As early as that first pregnancy test, many women begin to feel the stirrings of a protective mother waking within them. This is the primal part of us that is designed to keep our baby safe and thriving in the womb, that continues to protect our little one when they join us in the world, and that relies heavily on intuition. Observe any mother animal in the wild and you will see that she does not hesitate to protect her young at the first inkling of danger.

> Resonance is the art of embodying the feminine. However you feel in the moment is how you proceed. It's based on resonance, not on how it looks or how it's supposed to be.
>
> —ROCHELLE SCHIECK

IS SHYNESS OR SHAME INHIBITING YOUR INTUITION?

Trusting yourself relies on nurturing your relationship to your inner knowing. You do this through slowing down and getting quiet, dropping into your body through conscious movement and touch practices, and honoring gut feelings when they arise. Conveniently, pregnancy gives you infinite opportunities to play around with these techniques. As you bring your attention to your intuition and really begin to see that often you do know what's best for you and your baby, notice if you can recognize when it's more challenging to tap into that deep and steady part of yourself. Many moms-to-be say that they feel shy, embarrassed, or even ashamed to express these hits of intuition to those around them, and they begin questioning their gut feelings. When these thoughts come up, they can fill you with doubt about the messages you're receiving. If you go out to dinner and order a steak well done and it comes out rare, you may think, *I don't want to be difficult, maybe it's not that bad, I should probably just eat it instead of sending it back*. Or if you tell your OB that you are hoping for an unmedicated birth or a delayed cord cutting and they dismiss your request or make you feel silly or uninformed, you may defer to their point of view, discounting your own intuition. Or you may share a vulnerable feeling with a friend or family member only to receive a strong and contradictory opinion in return, leaving you questioning the felt sense in your heart. This ongoing doubt can damage the line of communication between you and your intuition; before you know it, you find yourself pushing down your true sense of knowing. Do this over and over and you will be cut off from who you really are, but with some simple curiosity and awareness (noticing when you disregard these signals from within), you can shape your intuition into a trustworthy tool that will guide you through pregnancy and birth.

Intuition is present-moment information. It's a feeling that you instantly experience when faced with a person, place, thing, or circumstance. Many people experience intuition or resonance through their physicality. When you meet the midwife who will be at your birth, do you feel an openness around your heart? Does your throat feel clenched? Or does your belly flip-flop? Others experience resonance or intuition in colors or images. Notice what you see when your doula comes into the room—flashes of fields of flowers or dark storm clouds offer very different sets of information. There is no right way to tap into your intuition, and in the early days of practice, you may not feel or see anything at all. Don't give up! It can be empowering to notice the resonance you feel at pivotal choice points throughout the day. Notice how you feel when you meet someone new, or when you are walking somewhere you have never been before. Under that feeling is information that you can use to make good decisions. Conversely, notice how you feel the next time you receive a hit of intuition or a gut instinct, and you *don't* honor it. Luckily, you will have the opportunity to make a different choice the next time you receive a tap from your intuition. The more you listen to your gut feelings, the stronger they become. Eventually, you can live your whole life being guided by this knowing part of yourself.

Fortify Your Force Field

As you spend more time honing this connection to your gut feelings, noticing resonance, and pivoting accordingly, you may find yourself becoming protective of this inner guidance system, avoiding anything, or anyone, that will knock you off your center and disrupt your connection to your intuition GPS. This is a good thing. Just as you are bringing awareness to all the things you consume during pregnancy—food, media, books, and TV—you can stretch this to include ideas, opinions, advice, and guidance offered from others, only letting in the helpful stuff and keeping what's not helpful out. Doula and women's mentor Khefri Riley calls this protective state a "bubble of peace," an invisible energetic force field that allows you to keep out what doesn't support you and to let in what does. "You have the power to consciously create your pregnancy, birth, and postpartum experience, and one way to do it is to build a force field around you, a protective energetic field that surrounds you," she explains. Some expecting mothers consciously move into this protective bubble as soon as they sense fear or negativity coming at them. "I stepped into a rose gold bubble that kept out fearful statistics about advanced maternal age," says Alissa Moreno, who had her third baby a month shy of her forty-fourth birthday. "I asked myself, 'Is this information going to help me or not?' And if a medical professional seemed anxious about something having to do with my pregnancy or birth plan or about a choice I was making, I let them hold the fear."

From an energetic point of view, creating a porous force field (where you let in what you want to let in) around you will help you remain in the calm, open state of mind that is essential for an easeful pregnancy and a smooth birth experience. One of your superpowers as a pregnant person is this self-generated boundary between you and the rest of the world—even with your partner, family, and friends, and especially with anyone in the medical system. Feel it vibrating subtly around you at all times, keeping out mental and emotional disturbances that feed fear, anxiety, and negativity. You have the ability to protect yourself and keep the channels that link you to your intuition wide open and unfettered by outside noise.

> Pregnancy, postpartum, and birth are profound times to awaken your own inner sovereignty and center yourself in the field of all possibilities. You have to imagine all possibilities because you want the highest possible outcome.
>
> —KHEFRI RILEY

They're Your Feelings, Not Your Baby's

You can also use your force field to keep your own feelings in check so they don't leak into your baby's realm. Imagine constructing a barrier between outsized emotions that may be temporarily wreaking havoc in your mind and your baby's safe space in your womb. Tell your little one that fear, anxiety, and so on are your feelings and that you are managing them and they do not have to take them on. You might say, "I'm fine, you're fine. I love you. It's OK. We're going to be OK."

Seek Out Good Stories

As you move through your pregnancy and get closer to giving birth, notice the tenor of the birth stories that you are taking in. If you are only reading and listening to challenging stories, you will be working against developing the positive mindset that will be invaluable during the last weeks of pregnancy, throughout birth, and into the wild first months of motherhood. On the other hand, taking in empowering birth stories, told from real women, can have a dramatic influence on your strength and belief in your abilities to bring this baby into the world. Positive doesn't mean sugar-coated, but it does mean uplifting and inspiring. It's so important to learn from the women who came before you. You may discover a new breathing practice or see firsthand that it's possible to have a beautiful, low-intervention birth, or learn about what a midwife or doula can do. If someone tries to tell you a difficult birth story, lovingly set a boundary with them—throw up that force field. Stop them and gently say, "This story doesn't serve me. Do you have a different one you can share?"

What If Things Go Right?

When you lean deeper into your intuition, you're actually leaning deeper into who you really are. You may feel overwhelmed, anxious, or unsure of what route to take, but you are so much bigger than those feelings. Pregnancy is designed for you to recognize how big you really are; you are expanding physically, yes, but you also have an opportunity to expand emotionally and energetically. It's in this bigger space, set behind worrisome thoughts, that you find the part of yourself that is brave, capable, and free. This is the part of yourself that believes in your abilities and knows that you are so much more than the constricted, limited, and anxious currents that move through you. Touch into this open optimism and you're activating the goddess within you, connected to an ancient lineage of pregnant and birthing women who came before you, guiding you to try something new, make a bold choice, and stand steadfast by what feels right.

GET TO KNOW YOUR NEGATIVITY BIAS

When faced with a decision during pregnancy and birth, pause for a few breaths and ask yourself if you are making your choices based on all the things that could go wrong or are leaning into what could go right? Often we are unaware of our negativity bias, installed deep in our DNA to protect us from harm. Take a moment to notice if you are inviting in a positive experience with an open, receptive state of being or if you are steeling yourself against a disastrous outcome, putting up your armor, shutting down, and backing away from an imagined danger. Begin to recognize how inhabiting a place of fear sparks your need to control the situation: Suddenly you're uptight and constricted, the opposite of the relaxed open state that leads you to a more easeful birth experience.

> There is such a small percentage of things that can go wrong in pregnancy and birth. If they do, it's devastating and it's awful, but we don't need to speak to that as the first point of entry. Let's speak instead to the possibility that things will go right and that listening to yourself can actually give you a huge amount of information to guide you through the process.
>
> —LAUREN CURTAIN, *women's health acupuncturist*

Nature's Offering

When you feel yourself disconnected from your intuition, there are simple ways to plug back into that place of knowing. "Be out in nature as much as you can and make sure you stop to feel your feet on Mother Earth," advises Ulrike Remlein. "Being grounded on Mother Earth is a primary way to feel grounded and trust in something that is much bigger than the chattering thoughts, passing stresses, and mundane concerns that can so easily rock you." You can take a hike or a walk around the park or in the neighborhood; you can garden, swim in a river or lake, or walk barefoot in the grass. Being in nature reminds you that you are part of something that is so much bigger than you and that is forever creating and changing.

You also don't have to look beyond yourself to find that reconnection to deep wisdom and guidance. The womb is the center of power (every person on Earth comes from a womb) and your source of creativity and unending trust. "I think of the womb as the very original computer," says Khefri. "The tissues of the womb are very similar to the tissues of the heart and brain—we have this cellular intelligence within us. Within the womb space, millions of cells are generated to create a baby. It's unfathomable—a space of complete and utter intelligence. If we look at it in that way, we have access to every single piece of information that we need; so I teach womb meditations, coming into stillness of the womb, and bringing awareness to the lower triangle of the body so women can access that power."

Outside of menstrual cramps and some basic pregnancy anatomy, many women may not even know they have a womb, feeling cut off, ashamed, or even numb around this area of their body. Spending time appreciating and acknowledging the power of your womb—it's growing a human being, remember?—helps build belief in yourself and encourage self-trust. To open the connection to your womb, simply place your hands on your lower abdomen and gently pour love into the womb and into the baby within. "Love heals everything," says Ulrike. Feel that love and then allow yourself to be in awe of the creative power coursing through you. Maybe you'll find yourself whispering—or shouting!—*if I can create this, then I can do anything!*

When an Older Pregnancy Is the Right Pregnancy

If you're pregnant and thirty-five or older, some care providers will consider you to be of "advanced maternal age." (Or worse, "geriatric"!) The thinking is that you are at greater risk for certain conditions or complications that could put you or your baby at risk. If you're working with a provider that is emphasizing your age, you know all about their concerns. But what about the other side of having babies a bit later in life? Women in their late thirties and forties have often lived full lives, are financially independent, more self-aware, comfortable with their relationship status, more mature, and increasingly capable of caring for others. "There's a strength that comes with age and an element of empowerment," says Jenny. "You're more conscious, more aware, more confident, and you can deeply savor the experience."

Hearing your intuition and following its direction is not always easy. There will be moments when you are too tired, too overwhelmed, too confused, too intimidated, or too ashamed to speak your truth. When they occur, draw deeper from the well of your own wisdom. The inner guidance you receive exists to protect you and your baby, and to teach him or her as well. By finding the courage to trust yourself, even when nobody else does, you are modeling self-trust for your child. So just give it a try. When you feel nervous, worried, doubting, and unstable, lean into the love you have for your baby—and let that love help you find the fortitude to take on anything, or anyone, that dares to question your knowing, no matter how impressive their bearing may be. In so doing, you claim your mothering crown.

THE GIFT OF

INTIMACY

THE FIRST THREE treasures have taken you on an inward journey to discovering how stillness can be an entry point for opening and relaxing, to befriending your body and allying with its awesome capabilities, and to sinking into your center of self-trust and the wisdom of your womb. From this empowered place, you now open your arms outward to receive—because while this is your personal journey, you're not supposed to walk it all alone! In yet another paradox of pregnancy and mothering, while you could soldier on and attempt to tend to your ever-changing body and slip-sliding emotions on your own, you're actually designed to be held by others.

Pregnancy's path is not without twists and turns and moments that can rock your sure footing. You will experience weird shifts in your physicality, puffy parts that were never puffy before, strange aches and pains, or odd discharges that can leave you embarrassed and wondering if this or that is "normal" or even safe for you and your baby. And nobody prepares you for all the emotional stuff that is coming to the surface. You may bump up against old stories that you thought were gone for good—questions around your ability to give birth or to be a great parent. There may be days when you wonder how the primal act of procreation, which has been happening since the beginning of time, can be rife with so much uncertainty. "During pregnancy, women are walking a labyrinth of being mortal, becoming immortal, and coming back to mortal," says master doula Haize Hawke. "That's an incredible tightrope walk. It can be transformational or it can be terrifying if you don't have a support system in place."

Real intimacy is in short supply in our modern world. So many of us live away from family and dear friends, and rely more than we realize on hits of connection by screen and social media. But pregnancy, by the nature of its sheer creative force that hurtles you from one version of yourself into another, demands the fortification of genuine human connection. As our first insight, Treat Yourself Gently (page 35), teaches, pregnant women must be seen and held by others. The positive impact of having your thoughts, concerns, fears, and hopes received by another human being cannot be measured. It's as vital as staying hydrated, eating fresh and vibrant foods, and regularly resting.

It may seem deceptively simple, but there is an almost magical alchemy that takes place when an expecting mother feels safe to open her heart to another. Pregnancy is a deeply emotional time that can bring up a lot, perhaps more than you bargained for when signing the invisible contract to become a parent, or parent again. You may be working against unattended traumas from your childhood, your birth, or even those passed down from your maternal line. You may feel waves of fear, shame, confusion, or overwhelm. Giving voice to them is one of the most effective ways to bring these feelings up to the surface so they can move through you rather than burying themselves deeper into your heart and psyche. Sometimes the simple act of speaking can vaporize cycles of self-doubt. Sharing in a safe space, with at least one trusted person, is also a gateway into a deeper understanding of yourself. "When we talk without being interrupted we learn so much about ourselves—especially if we know somebody is really listening and not judging," says Davi Khalsa. "It makes us willing to share our deepest feelings."

These bursts of intimate connection are a vital part of a healthy, empowered, and meaningful pregnancy and can take many shapes. You may find the support you need through the kind, gentle eyes of your midwife or doula, a friend, or a family member. They may support you as you work through a frightening emotion or offer you a way out of the loneliness that can infiltrate pregnancy even when surrounded by people. Other times you may simply need a boost—a cheerleader to remind you that even though you waddle when you walk, even though you snapped at your partner four times before noon, and even though you haven't done laundry in weeks, you are doing great.

In Treasure Three, you created a force field to keep out negative energies and to support your building of self-trust, but now your task is to create an outlet for your fears and worries. Keep them to yourself and they will bounce against the container of your isolation and become stronger, but when challenging thoughts are vented through an escape hatch, they lose their potency and can move more easily through you. If opening like this feels like shaky new territory, remember that pregnancy is all about expansion—at your waistline as your body morphs to accommodate your growing baby, in your heart as you find more love in which to envelop the new member of your family, and in your mind as you take in ideas and information that support you along the path to motherhood. You are continually

> When we gather together and share our stories, share our sweet medicine during our pregnancies, and process them in postpartum, we create an interconnected space to heal one another, and in doing so, heal our future generations.
>
> —KHEFRI RILEY

pushing past your comfort zone and discovering new ways of being along the way. So many of us are operating at peak levels of independence, wearing our ability to go it alone like some deranged badge of honor. For many women, asking for help, or even admitting a need, has become an act of bold vulnerability. After all, doing it "all" has become an expected part of modern womanhood, but expanding your circle past your own abilities, and even the care of your partner, can buoy you in immeasurable ways.

"In the West, everybody's so fiercely independent, but women do need that circle of support," says Robin Lim from her clinic in Bali. "I know women here sometimes envy that independence, but what they have instead is real community." As you call in your support team, keep in mind that the people who will fortify you during pregnancy are not the advice givers, overtalkers, or know-it-alls. They are the gracious ones who make space for you to be whatever you really are, and to feel whatever you're truly feeling, in any given moment. These are the people who reflect your feminine force and knowing; they believe in your abilities and trust that even when you feel lost, confused, or overwhelmed, you will find your way to the direction that is best for you and your baby. During pregnancy, there is an opportunity for a very special type of connection—it can change you for life.

Who's on Your Team?

Your support team begins with your prenatal care providers, the folks who will be guiding you through pregnancy and birth. The people who you choose to usher you through this amazingly important time in your life will have a major impact on your experience. At this point you are likely working with one or more care providers—an OB who will support you to deliver in a hospital, or a home birth or birth center midwife, or one of the many combinations of both. Depending on the shape of your family, you may be partnered with someone who is hoping for a different care experience than the one that you are looking for.

There are many ways to form a pregnancy and birth support team. Deciding on your team—this is likely a doctor or midwife, or a midwifery group, in combination with a doula—is an essential first step in your pregnancy experience. They will be the ones who will support you in bringing your baby safely into the world, and you will be thrust into an incredibly intimate relationship with them, imparting a massive amount of trust into their wisdom and expertise. To facilitate an experience that feels right to you, it's important to partner with care providers who are aligned with your personal approach and philosophy and who support any specific needs and desires that you may have. You may feel passionate about unmedicated birth, delayed cord cutting, or an epidural-supported birth experience. You may feel clear that you want minimal diagnostic tests during pregnancy, or a water birth, or a recovery night or two at the hospital after your baby arrives.

> The most important message our midwives give to mothers during pregnancy is, "We believe in you."
>
> —ROBIN LIM

Many Ways to Birth

With her first baby, my co-author Marisa compromised with her then husband and worked with a team of midwives who delivered in a hospital. This gave them both the comfort they were looking for. My coauthor Amely worked with a group of midwives at a birthing center, but labored first at home. Our photographer Jenny had to take a different path, undergoing a conscious C-section for safety precautions. My first child arrived in a water birth at a hospital with my excellent midwife Hilary, and my second two were born at home with my trusted midwife Davi. My treasured doula, Khefri, was there for the first two births—she missed the second one by a hair as I delivered in under three hours! Though our births were different, we were each supported by a circle of care that helped us feel tended to and empowered.

Whether you partner with a midwife or OB, this is the time to connect to yourself, trust, and make the effort to find the care provider(s) who reflect your choices. The best prenatal care is rooted in shared decision-making. This means that your care providers will give you clear information about the risks and benefits of any test or procedure and will then honor and support the decisions you make for yourself and your baby. They will make space for you to openly share your thoughts and feelings at every step of the process. In this way, you are truly partnering with your team, each of you dedicated to creating the most supportive and successful pregnancy and birth experience. "Our role is to support the journey they are on," says Davi, who has twenty years of midwifery practice under her belt. "I feel the midwife's most important job is to let the woman speak, to hear how she's feeling and ask her questions. It is so important for people to be heard."

While there is no wrong way to receive prenatal support, the midwifery model is based on centuries of woman-to-woman care. Midwives will always do an assessment to ensure that an expecting mother is not high risk and to understand her specific needs or concerns. "If you have any preferences or you know things that you do or don't want to happen in your childbirth experience, we want you to be able to drop your shyness enough to share it with us," says Robin Lim. "We always look in the mother's eyes and say, 'We'd like to hear from you.'" But for some, the ability to choose a prenatal care team is a luxury. Geographic location or resources may leave a pregnant person with limited options. If you feel that your provider is unable to provide you with the level of attention or care that you are hoping for, there are other ways to create an elevated, supported pregnancy and birth. If it is within your budget, you can hire a doula—a care provider whose primary job is to ensure that you feel safe, heard, and supported throughout the birthing process. Or you may enlist another trusted person from your friends or family group to be your primary source of support. (This may require that they do some reading up on what happens during pregnancy and birth and how to best be there for you through it all.) Or you can find solace, wisdom, and guidance from the endless resources available online and in books and podcasts. Either way, you can play a big part in getting the pregnancy and birth experience you are hoping for by being thoroughly educated and by understanding your rights. "I was my own best detective," says mom Jenny. "I would get as informed as possible and then find professionals who could respond to my concerns—and then I'd see if their responses matched my own point of view or intuitive hit."

> My daughter sends her midwives flowers on her birthday every year. She feels gratitude because she knows that I had an incredible birth experience, therefore, *she* had an incredible birth experience.
>
> —ROBIN LIM

Build Your Village

If it takes a village to raise a child, it also takes a village to support a mama during pregnancy and through the gateway into motherhood. Having extra hands to do simple chores, make food, tend to older children, or hold the baby so she can shower or nap is an essential element of postpartum care found in cultures around the world. Receiving this level of external support can be invaluable when you are sleep deprived, hormonal, lactating, and hungry, yet there is another level of new mother support that may be even more important. When even one person takes a few moments to stop, look a new mother in the eye, and ask her how she is feeling, the impact on her mental and emotional well-being can be profound.

In *The First Forty Days*, we encourage an expecting mother to build her support team before baby arrives, at least in the third trimester. And in writing this book, we stand by that guidance, but this time our hope is that she has a circle around her that will be there for her from the uncertain early weeks of pregnancy all the way through the early weeks of motherhood. This is a key aspect of treating yourself gently. (Flip back to the four insights, beginning on page 35, and remind yourself about this essential part of a supported pregnancy.) This can be even one trusted friend who will meet you exactly where you are and tip the scales to your needs, so your load of obligation gets lightened whenever possible. The wisely chosen members of your village do not expect to be hosted, tended to, or emotionally supported. They are there for you in whatever state you may be inhabiting that day—irritable, worried, joyful, achy, or hopeful. You will never have to erect a protective facade when you're with these people, and you will not have to meet any expectations.

> Psychologically, it's becoming really apparent that we are missing that village. A lot of women are working as if they're not pregnant, carrying on all the same duties. There is not a lot of taking care of the woman when pregnant. The fact is, it's a special time, you are growing a human being and should not be expected to do so much! What would it be like if the pregnant woman had sisters, cousins, and friends taking care of *her*?
>
> —LAUREN CURTAIN

Sometimes You Need a Pro

The power of a pair of great listening ears cannot be measured, but there may be moments in your pregnancy that require more than what a good friend can provide. Throughout your pregnancy, and especially in the first trimester, you may find yourself traversing shaky, unfamiliar ground, and feel hesitant or unsure about sharing difficult feelings. The early weeks of pregnancy can be an especially delicate time. You are undergoing a massive transformation physically and emotionally, but to the rest of the world, these changes are still invisible. You are moving around town with the entire universe within you, yet nobody will get up to give you a seat on the subway—it can be jarring and confusing! If you are waiting until the start of the second trimester to share your baby news, you may feel even more isolated and alone as complicated or worrisome thoughts zip around your mind, and your heart feels elated one moment and like a sack of lead bricks in another. "Pregnancy can be hard, and women may not be able to talk about it," says Lauren Curtain. "A lot of women won't even tell friends how they're feeling; they don't want to burden them or bother them. They are going through this alone, which is really sad. Having a trusted care provider or another caring professional will give them support and a place to vocalize how they're feeling. This is essential all through pregnancy, but especially in the first trimester."

> We're so desperate to find that container of caring, like-minded people who say, "Yeah, I'm with you on this journey."
>
> —ROCHELLE SCHIECK

In addition to first-trimester jitters, pregnancy can bring up a range of deep and complex feelings. As you expand to bring new life into the world, you are opening up in new ways too. In exploring Treasure Three, you may have noticed that your sensitivity and intuition are buzzing—your pregnancy superpowers. But seated right next to them can be a handful of feelings that may seem bigger than you. Pregnancy is a major initiation and can stir up fears or unresolved trauma. Getting pregnant may have been extremely challenging; if so, now that you've arrived, it might be difficult to relax into the experience. You may have chosen to have a baby on your own and are wondering if you have made the right decision. You may have questions about your partnership and how the two of you will be as parents. Maybe you have challenges with your mother and are wondering if your child is going to feel the same way about you. You may have terminated one or more pregnancies and are feeling the significance of choosing to move forward now. Or you may have experienced loss and feel concerned about the safe unfolding of this pregnancy. If any of these dilemmas starts to cause significant distress, it's wise to seek experienced support from a therapist, counselor, or spiritual mentor (or even a somatic-based therapist, where the focus is more on feeling than talking)—not so much for them to fix anything but, as Lauren explains, "to help you come to your own realization of your truth by hearing you deeply."

The harder emotions that come up during pregnancy may be difficult to name, defying simple categorization like "scared to give birth" or "worried about how we'll afford a child." This is because being pregnant can be like discovering a hidden door that leads to an unexplored chamber below your house. This place is part of you, but it's dark and intimidating. This is where your unconscious fears and unresolved traumas are stored—trauma from your own birth or childhood or sexual trauma. These currents may stem from your own history or may be something that you have carried down from your family line.

If you're feeling bold, you may choose to shine a light into the dusty corners of this subterranean room, understanding that bringing these shadows into the light of awareness is the only way to heal them. A desire to heal is the first and most courageous step, and from there it's good to seek professional guidance. This is work that is best done with the skilled support of a trauma-informed therapist or counselor, who can help you navigate overwhelming feelings. "If it feels frightening to be pregnant, or if many unpleasant things are coming up, it might be wise to work with someone who can guide you within to release trauma," says Ulrike Remlein, who supports women in healing the innermost aspects of themselves. "You need someone who has a spiritual background and sees that a human being is not just the body, some emotions, and some thoughts, but a spiritual being having a human experience."

> We know it's wise to bring in a little extra help when a woman has a fear that seems like it's got a lot of emphasis—when it is really big for her.
> —DAVI KHALSA

When confronting hard emotions, ideally you will be receiving support on a variety of levels: sharing with trusted friend(s) and working with a professional therapist or counselor. You do not have to do it alone. When attending to these deeper, most tender parts of yourself, the idea is to support the feelings in moving

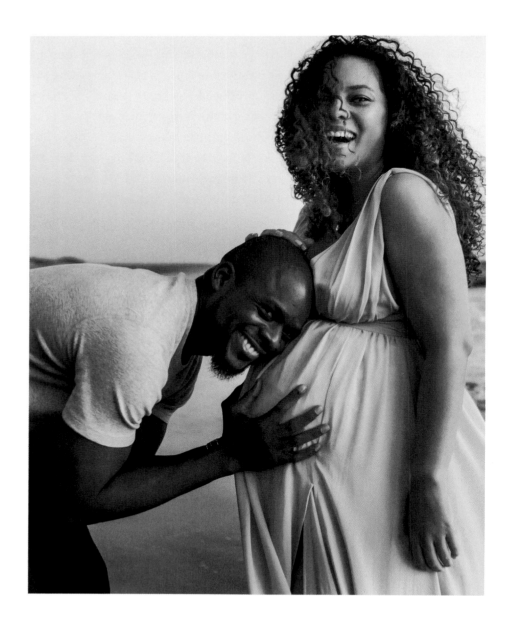

up and out. Trauma is stored in the body, so movement of any kind can be a wonderful addition to therapy or counseling. Yoga, dance, walking, and swimming, or body-oriented care such as gentle chiropractic, cranial sacral, Reiki, and massage—these are all wonderful ways to support the release of challenging feelings and emotions. "Anything that supports being relaxed and present in the body is what we want to do," says Ulrike.

Journaling can also help create a space for the harder feelings to move out of you. Open up a blank page and just let it rip—write like nobody's watching, because nobody is. This is your safe space to express yourself totally and completely. Give yourself the challenge of opening up, uncensored and uninhibited. Write, sketch, scribble— just get it out. Maybe you give three pages to writing "AHHHHHHHHHHHH!" in all caps. As you write, notice when feelings of shame bubble up. Shame is a trickster emotion, sneaking up when you least expect it and blocking your ability to experience the depth of your emotions. If you are ashamed that you have worries about being a good mother, you won't be able to address the heart of those worries and begin to dissolve them. Shame is completely natural, and acknowledging when you're feeling ashamed is an effective way to move through those feelings so you can get to what's underneath. Also note when you're judging yourself.

Intimacy and Your Partner

The village that you gather around you—any combination of your midwife, OB, doula, friends, family, and therapist—is there to hold you up as you move through pregnancy and into birth. But the benefits of this care will also radiate past your own heart and into your primary relationship. Having a trusted group of people that you can turn to can free up space within your relationship with your partner, giving you room to keep your dynamic deep, connected, and fulfilling. Amazing things happen when you don't expect your partner to be everything to you at all times. Pregnancy is actually a beautiful time to deepen in intimacy with your partner. While you certainly may not feel like stepping into a sexual space all the time with your morphing body and swinging hormones, there are many ways to remain close during pregnancy, staying lovers while you move toward becoming parents.

For partners, genuine intimacy happens when they understand that holding a pregnant person is a big responsibility! Some days your partner may feel like they can do no right. It will help if they understand the nature of pregnancy. Guide them to read the section on naturally amplified vata (page 36), which creates changeability, anxiety, and sometimes irritability for the pregnant one. Then gently suggest they approach you as they would changing weather and seasons—prepared, but not attached to how it will be, and not taking the inclement moments personally.

Sometimes, like it or loathe it, during (inevitable) relationship challenges, the best move is to simply defer to the expecting parent. "During pregnancy, I tell the dads, mom is always right!" says Davi Khalsa, noting that sensitivity increases and concerns about how the future will be or how finances will work may heighten, and arguing every point logically is not always helpful. Sometimes the best thing the partner can do is, "Put your arms around her and say, Honey—we'll always find a way."

A Simple Intimacy Practice

Siddhi Ellinghoven recommends this easy practice for partners at every stage of the pregnancy journey—from conception onward. "Intimacy means 'into me you see,'" she says. "If a couple does this in the morning, they will be connected all day."

- Sit knee to knee with your partner. Take their hands in yours, resting hands on knees.

- Gaze into each other's eyes for four minutes. If you feel inclined to giggle, talk, look away, or squirm, simply breathe and get curious—can you stay connected? And what does it feel like after you pass through the awkwardness?

- If you like, you may join hands in lotus mudra. Each person places their hands together in prayer position; keeping the base of the hands together, and thumbs and little fingers touching, allow the index, middle, and ring fingers to open like a lotus flower blossoming. Link your pinkie fingers with theirs.

While the pregnant person deserves extra care and reverence, building connection during pregnancy is still a two-way street. You can support your partner in supporting you by remembering that they are not a mind reader. Make things easier by opening up to them about what's going on for you. Bring them into your world by sharing how you are feeling emotionally and physically; let them know what's changing for you. It can help to tap into some compassion for what it could feel like to be observing you during pregnancy; to be outside of the experience. This is their baby too, yet they don't know what it feels like to carry the child inside of them. Can you welcome them into your experience? As you experiment with opening up to your partner, do so with discernment. Oversharing may add too much pressure and put unnecessary weight on your dynamic. Remember, your support team is there for the nitty-gritty stuff. Can you lighten the load between you and your partner, without diluting the essence of what you're feeling? If you are working through harder feelings, it may help to tell them that you will be leaning on outside support so you don't put too much on your relationship.

> Make sure you have a caregiver who makes you feel heard and respects your voice. Everything a pregnant person says is sacred and should be respected as such.
>
> —KHEFRI RILEY

Pregnancy is also the time to check in with your partner to see how they're feeling about adding another member to the family. It's good to take the time during pregnancy to ask each other some key logistical questions about how life will look in the early months caring for a brand-new infant. Now is also the time to create some space to really hear what's going on for your partner as they prepare to become a parent, or a parent again. They will have their own hopes, concerns, and fears. Can you make some time to really listen to what's happening for them?

Inevitably, you and your partner will hit some bumps along the road to parenthood. Our friend and wise one Damian Hagglund learned during his wife's pregnancy how resolving conflicts as soon as possible did wonders to help her remain in a balanced, harmonious state. "From my perspective as an Ayurvedic practitioner, holding anything in heats up the body and increases cortisol levels, which is not helpful for the baby in utero. Knowing this, when things came up, I would stop everything, connect eye to eye, and sort it out immediately. We found that physical intimacy was key: holding hands while we spoke, as well as communicating in a softer way than normal, and owning my part in any conflict. Simply owning it would take away a lot of the problems."

ENCIRCLED AFTER LOSS

Kati Greaney faced what is quite possibly the hardest and most excruciating, and typically invisible, part of the pregnancy experience—profound loss. But through turning to her circle of intimate support, she was able to step through the pain and heal.

I was really empowered when I was pregnant with my second child, Cedar. While we were on our farm in Utah that summer, I was shoveling and lifting. Everybody always got such a kick out of me because I was this big pregnant woman doing all the physical work. I had it in my head that women all over the world do this; they don't stop their whole life when they're pregnant, and so I just kept doing everything.

I felt pretty good, though it was difficult also caring for my two-and-a-half-year-old, Jorro. He was kind of threatened by the new baby and very challenging. After the summer in Utah, I had a small baby blessing. Three girlfriends came over and we made little potions and a necklace for me to wear during my birth, and I remember when they were painting my belly I felt like Cedar hadn't moved in a while. One of my friends is a midwife, and when she couldn't find his heartbeat, I tried to stay in a festive mood, but made an appointment with my midwife for the next day.

The next morning at the appointment, everything was in slow motion. I remember my husband Pete making small talk with the midwife, and me feeling like, I need to hear this heartbeat right away, right away, right away. And they couldn't find it. They hooked me up to another machine and they still couldn't find it. At the hospital, nobody was telling me what was going on. I was scanning everyone's faces for information. I really didn't think that there was a possibility that the baby had died. Finally, the doctor told us that they couldn't find the heartbeat and I just went into shock.

They said they needed to induce me right away, but luckily my midwife was there to say that's not the case. She told me that I needed to take this information and process it. That was a huge gift to me because I was able to take the time to digest the information first. I went to the river. I gathered with my female friends, we made a fire, and I began to understand what was being asked of me. Eventually I got to a place where I said, "Okay, I can do this." I went into the hospital the next day and was able to be fully present for the delivery. This made it a very powerful, even transformative experience.

When they handed him to me, I screamed. It was the sound that mothers make when they lose a child, it's a very specific pitch, a sound that I've never made before. It just came through me; it was a universal frequency and I could feel it connected me through time and space. I remember coming home from the hospital and feeling like I needed to have another baby right away, but I knew that I had to wait. I went on this whole healing journey and finally arrived at a place where I was ready for another baby in a different way, not just to fill a void.

On the anniversary of what would have been Cedar's first birthday, I was pregnant again, but when I went in for the first checkup, they couldn't find the heartbeat. I just kept going and then a couple months later I was pregnant again and began the journey of being pregnant after going through loss; that's a really different type of pregnancy. I kept feeling that at every step of the way the baby was going to die, and I had to tell myself, "This is a different story, this is a different baby." She came very quickly. It was amazing to be able to listen to my body and have this process with her, and when they handed her to me, that same noise came out through me, but it was different. Jasmine looked exactly like Cedar, and it was just so beautiful and triumphant, but also painful and full of so much memory. Now we're a family of four, but we're really a family of five. We have this other presence that's always with us in beautiful and hard ways.

> People think that grief shrinks over time, but we grow around our grief.
>
> —DR. LOIS TONKIN,
> *researcher on loss and grief*

In addition to her intimate circle of friends and family, Kati received immense support from HAND of the Bay Area (handsupport.org), an organization offering support after the loss of a baby, before, during, or after birth.

Facing Loss, Together

Allowing intimacy with others is also a way to layer in support should the unthinkable occur. If you have ever experienced a pregnancy loss, you have likely been thrown into a swirling sea of emotions, navigating waves of grief, emptiness, disappointment, heartbreak, and even guilt and shame. The onslaught of feelings can threaten to unhinge you from yourself indefinitely, leaving you to question if you will ever feel like yourself again. When faced with such grief, it can feel overwhelming to take a step in any direction. Walking the labyrinth of pregnancy means knowing anything is possible. Should things take a difficult turn, the first thing to do is nothing at all. Give yourself as much time as you need to grieve. And while the healing of your heart is a very personal process, grief is a path that is designed to be traversed with others. This is a tender, raw, and vulnerable space to inhabit, but if you can allow others to hold you during this time, it will help to mend the fractured places inside you. Open yourself up to the care of trusted friends and family, support groups, or therapy (or all three). "Sharing and being witnessed was hugely important to my healing," says Kati Greaney, who lost her second baby close to the due date (see Kati's story on pages 110–111). "I joined circles with women who had experienced similar loss. Other women were sharing their experiences, and I felt so seen. I remember one woman saying, 'I will never go to a baby shower again, I will never be happy for another pregnant woman again,' and I was just like, *Hallelujah, thank you*. I've never felt permission to say that."

> When we are dealing with birth, we are also dealing with death. We are dealing with opposites. It's really confronting to women to face that reality, that something could go wrong. How do you process it? How do you go from highest of highs to lowest of lows?
>
> —LAUREN CURTAIN

There is never a more important time to let yourself be loved by others. "For me, it was really about the sisters," says Kati. "I never used that word 'sisters' before, but the women who gathered around me at this time were so much more than friends. This was the real sisterhood, like the ancient village. That was just so fundamental to me. I think that community is such a huge part of grieving, but so often in our culture, we do it in isolation and we feel really uncomfortable around it." Your care provider can also be a source of support during a time of grief. Master doula Haize Hawke works closely with her clients during the grieving process. "I help them first acknowledge that they had the baby and then I help them grieve," she says. "I help them grieve the baby and the life they thought they were going to have. We mourn that loss together. We do a lot of breath work to release any holding in the body, lots of meditation, Reiki, and journals with prompts that I give them. I do it with both the mother and the father because the partners go through it too. I let them both know it's okay to be sad, but help them understand that the sadness doesn't need to define you. You want it to move through you—and it's important to acknowledge that this child is still a part of the family. They have just gone over to the other side and are now an ancestor, which is very special."

You are not supposed to do it alone. As you move through your remaining months of pregnancy, and turn your sights to an empowered and uplifting birth, open your heart to those who want to help. Your vulnerability is a virtue and it will be held with tenderness by your chosen support team.

THE GIFT OF

POWER

YOU NOW HOLD four precious treasures within you, gems that sparkle and reflect the light, and that will hold you through the remaining days of your pregnancy, through birth, and into the first forty days of motherhood—and beyond. With Stillness you experience what it feels like to slow down, get quiet, and really hear yourself. Honor brings you back to a place of wonder and awe for all that your body can do. Trust connects you to an unwavering source of belief in who you are and what you (and your baby) need to feel safe and comfortable, and Intimacy lifts you up with an unwavering circle of support. Each treasure shines brightly when practiced on its own, but they come to their fullest expression when they build upon each other, one leading you to the next along the course of your pregnancy and to your moment of birth, where your final treasure reveals itself—Power.

If you're reading this during the final weeks of pregnancy, you may be feeling a lot of things, but powerful likely isn't one of them. At this stage of the process, your baby is growing about a half pound a week and is taking up quite a bit of space in a residence that was already tiny to begin with. You may be facing challenges that have been with you for most of pregnancy: constipation, indigestion, and lower back pain, and now you're experiencing the sprinkles on top of that discomfort sundae with hemorrhoids, reflux, nonstop peeing, and the phenomenon that wise woman extraordinaire Dr. Aviva Romm calls "lightning crotch." Achy, waddling, and simultaneously starving and stuffed, you may find it hard to believe that you'll be experiencing a profoundly empowering rite of passage in just weeks, or maybe even days.

The primal power and heart expansion that a woman experiences through the birth process is unlike anything else. Movies and TV have created one narrative about birth—often depicting a screaming woman who's overwhelmed, uncentered, in agony, and on the brink of disaster, only to be saved by a doctor who swoops in just in time to scream at her to "PUSH!" But that story's getting old, and modern birthing people are rewriting that script. Real people are posting raw, fiercely honest shares about their pregnancy and birth experiences, and in doing so, they are systematically replacing stale tropes about what it means to have a baby. The way birth looks is as diverse as the hundreds of thousands of people who do it every day, and a brave and growing group of mothers, parents, partners, care providers, and birth advocacy organizations are reminding us that the experience can be gentle, primal, beautiful, joyful, sensual, fierce, or focused. It can be all of these things, some of these things, or none of them at all.

Nurturing the Ninth Month

In these final weeks, Chinese medicine advises tender loving care for the Kidneys, the organ system that supports your reproductive power. This care looks like good sleep, no overexertion, nutrient-dense foods, and warm clothing. It's particularly important to keep your feet, knees, and back nice and warm to avoid pain in the lumbar spinal column. This may mean keeping your home warm if you live in a chilly climate or throwing on extra fuzzy socks and another sweater. It's a good idea to keep up with regular movement, but, as with the rest of your pregnancy, avoid pushing too hard.

As pregnant women continue to have greater access to real stories, and as they become increasingly educated about their rights in the birthing space, they are reclaiming birth and the impact a positive and supported birth experience can have on their life, and on their baby's life. Women are starting to wake up to the fact that there is no "right" or "wrong" way to birth; regardless of whether that birth was medicated or unmedicated, in a hospital or at home, or cesarean or vaginal. However you give birth, you will discover hidden reserves of strength and tap into a steely determination that will carry you through the ultimate moment of transformation, when you become a Mother or Mother Again. There is a fierceness that is ignited when you bring your baby from inside of you to the outside world—and it is a light that will never go out. However your birth unfolds, you will never feel the same way about yourself again. You will discover that all birth is sacred.

As women begin to recognize the significance of birth, not just as a medical procedure, but as an initiatory event with important implications for their own personal development, women can take back the power of birth that belongs to them and channel it into greater connection with their own evolution, the evolution of their children, and the healing of the planet through the creation of a more conscious society.

—ISA GUCCIARDI, PHD, *The New Return to the Great Mother*

ENTERING THE IN-BETWEEN

Along with many other ideas about birth, the concept of a "due date" is becoming *out*dated. Many care providers offer a loose idea of when labor may start so that expecting parents can manage their expectations and give their baby undisturbed space to arrive on their own timeline. Pregnancy seems to stretch on and on in the last weeks, but when you enter what Haize Hawke calls your "guess date window," which extends to two weeks before or two weeks after the day when labor could begin, you will have stepped into a very special space. She refers to this as the In-Between, a precious period where you have another chance to sit with the first four treasures and prepare your mindset for the threshold you will soon pass through. "It is important to drop into your most innermost thoughts, concerns, and worries and release any residue," she says. "Many months have been spent to prepare your body, mind, and spirit for the labor path, and sometimes a little can pop up again. Take this time to let go of any remaining fears. Take this time to love on yourself. Take the time to be with your partner in deep and meaningful ways." The In-Between is like a final deep exhale before you step into the birthing journey. This is your chance to recognize if there is anyone in your circle who is adding stress or discomfort to your life, perhaps by asking one too many times if baby will be coming soon or offering unsolicited thoughts on what you're eating or doing or not doing. Practice putting up your force field, only letting in what feels good and supportive. This is your last chance to get good at this before moving into birth and the postpartum period. "Anything that is stressful, any people that are stressing you out, offer you a great opportunity to form some boundaries that will support you postpartum," says Blyss Young, midwife and founder of Birthing Blyss Midwifery. "Focus on doing things that build oxytocin. Oxytocin is the initiator for labor so keep it calm, stress-free, and full of love. Do what makes you feel juicy: Go on a date with your honey, watch a comedy, have sex, watch a sunset, dance, hang out with girlfriends. Enjoy those moments before your new normal sets in."

There Is No Correct Way to Birth

One of the forces igniting this reawakening to the transformative power of birth is understanding and accepting that birth can be many things and it can look many ways. You choose your care providers and create a birth plan based on a variety of factors that may be different for each individual. These choices are based on economics, access to care, personal history, past traumas, specific medical needs, spiritual and philosophical beliefs, mental well-being, and much more. An expecting mother may choose to birth with an OB in her local hospital because that is what feels right to her or because that's what's available to her or because that's what her insurance will cover. Another may choose to give birth at home with a birthing tub, a midwife, and a doula. Yet another may birth in a birthing center, and there is now a small but vocal group of people in the freebirth community who are birthing their babies completely outside of the medical system. "I deeply believe in a woman's right to choose how she births," says birth advocate Lacey Haynes. "But what I believe in more than that is giving women the information and the lifelong learning, so that they choose to birth in a way that actually supports their long-term evolution and long-term satisfaction."

> It doesn't matter where you birth. You can birth in an alley. You can birth on the side of a mountain. You can birth in your home. You can birth in the hospital. You are going to birth that baby out of your body and once you take ownership that your body belongs to you, you will see that no matter where *you* birth, there *you* are.
>
> —KHEFRI RILEY

Sometimes a birth will take an unexpected turn and a woman who was hoping to have an unmedicated birth will have an emergency C-section. A home birth mother may have to be transferred to the hospital. A person planning on an epidural may deliver too fast to receive that intervention. Sometimes a pharmaceutical assistance like Pitocin will be critical. However, wherever, a baby is born is right and beautiful. No approach is better or worse than another as long as the mother feels seen, safe, and secure throughout the process. And the way birth is experienced and integrated will be different for each person because at its essence, birth is several things at once: a normal, everyday process and a major life event.

For some women, birthing their baby is a transformative, spiritual experience that pushes them out of their everyday reality into the realm of the magical and divine. For others, it is a test of their mental and physical fortitude, offering a significant sense of accomplishment. For others, birth can feel quite intimidating and overwhelming. As Angela Garbes writes in her book *Like a Mother*, "As a culture, we have no collective definition of 'safe' when it comes to bringing our children into this world. Do you feel safest in a hospital or in your home? Would you feel more secure giving birth in a rented blow-up tub in your living room or in your bed, on the sheets you sleep in every night? Or would you prefer a bed with nurses nearby, a sterile operating table? The answer is different for each of us. 'Safe' can be synonymous with all of these environments."

In connecting so deeply with birthing experts and mothers, and turning to our own birth experiences, we feel it is essential to clear up the fuzziness that surrounds the idea of "natural birth." For many, "natural birth" implies that a birthing person had an unmedicated, vaginal birth, and, for those in favor of that choice, birthing in this way is said to be the better way. For us, and for our team of wise ones, just as there is no right way to birth, there is no birth that is more natural than another. Angela Garbes sums it up concisely: "A baby born of its mother's body is natural, whether it's pushed through her vagina or pulled out of her uterus." A C-section can be a lifesaving operation for a mother and her baby, she explains, and for women who have medical challenges like uterine fibroids, a cesarean section can be the most natural and safest option.

If you find yourself having a birth experience that you did not expect, this is your time to activate the trust you have placed in your care providers and in the space that you have chosen to birth, and to trust in the unfolding of the process in general. "Trust in the universe, in the midwives or the hospital; they all want your baby to be safe," says Damian Hagglund. "Understand, this child has come with its own destiny; if this child is destined to be born with a C-section in a hospital because it is the safest way for it to be born, then trust in that. That's beautiful, that's magical too, that's the unique expression of the universe in that child. That child will come out however it will come out."

As far as duration goes, your labor may be long and drawn out and moving slowly, requiring mental fortitude and physical stamina. Or your birth experience may be unexpectedly fast, hurtling you from one stage to the next before you can find your center. However long or short the path from Expecting Mother to Mother (or Mother Again) may be, you will be asked to lean into the treasures you have cultivated along the way, once again trusting yourself, your body, and your support team. By using the forty-ish weeks of pregnancy to cultivate a mindset of surrender, openness, and curiosity, you will enter into your unique birth experience with a soft and receptive spirit, with faith that you are completely capable and that something incredibly special is about to unfold. "It's bittersweet; I enjoy pregnancy and don't want it to end, but have been excited to experience labor for a while now," said expecting mother Amanda Carney, just days before giving birth to her daughter, Penn. "It feels like a privilege to be able to go through it. I'm going to learn a lot!" Regardless of how your birth unfolds, it will become your story, and your family's—a personal mythology that will offer depth and meaning for the rest of your life, and the smaller details surrounding your baby's arrival may not matter as much as you think. "This child has its unique birth, made uniquely by the universe; they're going to be a unique person; there's nothing we or anyone can do about it," adds Damian.

Shakti: The Power That's Yours

When you give birth, you are moving through the pinnacle of the creation process. You are at the doorway between gestating and welcoming new life, and in order to fully walk through this space, you will be asked to access a resource of primal power that resides deep inside you. One term for this specific current of power is "Shakti." "Shakti is a universal principle of the creative force of the universe," explains Khefri Riley. "It's the term for the creator mother goddess, the primal force that exists within all of us. There are many ways to access it, but I believe that birth is one of the most potent ways to tap this transformative power of creation—and it doesn't matter if the birth is cesarean or vaginal, with candles in a birthing center or with no frills in a shack. Shakti is non-discriminatory, and everyone has it.

It's your birthright to be held in your pregnancy journey and birth powerfully.
—KHEFRI RILEY

We might think we don't have it or can't access it—or that this kind of power only comes to the person who has money for a midwife or special treatment—but it's available to everyone. It's the internal wealth of personal power."

Regardless of how you choose to birth, and how your birth unfolds, it is impossible to come out on the other side of this experience unchanged. Consciously or unconsciously, you have been building up to this moment for months; once your baby is in your arms, you will have crossed a threshold that will leave you inhabiting a new version of yourself. This transitioning from one way to another is mirrored in the physiological unfolding that occurs during labor. There is a phase in labor aptly called "transition" where the baby moves through the fully dilated cervix into the birthing canal. It may have taken hours, or even days, to get to this point—this is often where many women feel that they can't go on; this is the breaking point. At transition, the Maiden, the younger, less evolved and less dynamic version of you, is not strong enough for what you're being asked to do. This is the exact moment where a woman evolves from Maiden to Mother. The younger woman in her dies so that she can be reborn as a mother—a new, more capable version of herself with far more strength than she has ever known.

> I think giving birth is as enlightened as we can get.
>
> —SIDDHI ELLINGHOVEN

"In birth, we are looking for powerful, not comfortable," says Haize Hawke. "There is a point in labor where this statement needs to be said. It can make the difference from having the labor be five more hours to two hours. Most birthers will try to find a "comfortable position" and there isn't one. They are running from the sensation they don't like when that is exactly where they need to lean in. We all do this in life too. Running from things and people who are too intense. If you don't want it chasing you, turn and face it."

If you have ever been in the room with a person who's giving birth, you know that something very powerful is occurring. Regardless of your spiritual beliefs, it's hard to miss the significance of one human life bringing forth another. There is something almost magical taking place as a woman opens herself to this most magnificent act of creation. As she moves deeper into labor, with contractions intensifying and her heart expanding and readying itself to meet her child, it's as if she takes on a mystical quality. "During birth, you are the portal that opens between two worlds to allow a spirit to come through," explains doula and wise one, Lori Bregman. "During birth, as the portal (you) opens, your crown chakra (top of head) and root chakra (perineum) busts open, and all the other chakras in between as well, to allow this spirit to move through you. You will get labor shakes from all the hormones, but it's also serious energy being moved, cleared, and opened. When you are this open, you are one with spirit/God/the universe. You have direct access to a higher power, your intuition, and source energy. Tune in and follow it!"

Just as pregnancy offers you the opportunity to deepen your relationship with yourself and others and to access a reverence and trust for what your body can do—perhaps for the first time ever—birth offers you the opportunity to turn on the switch to your personal power, a switch that once on, never turns off. It doesn't matter if you have lived a life of questioning and uncertainty, if you have been hesitant, fearful, shy, or unassuming. Every single birthing person will be shuttled out of their comfort zone and given the chance to harness their personal power. "I remember coming out of birth feeling like if somebody ever tells you that you are not something, then after you give birth, you know that *you are everything*," says mom Kati Greaney.

> When doubt creeps in when pregnant, birthing, and as a new mom, you can trust that you know what you and your baby need more than anyone else. You have all the knowledge within because you are the power.
> —LORI BREGMAN

You Are Designed to Birth

During labor, you will be asked to go to new places of strength and fortitude, but you won't be doing it through sheer will alone. Your body will be leading the charge, with the uterus in the driver's seat. The uterus is a power organ, part of what Latham Thomas, founder of the online community Mama Glow, calls your "sacred anatomy." During pregnancy, the uterus expands from 500 to 1000 times its normal size, growing from about two ounces to up to two pounds, she explains. This makes it the largest muscle of the body and the most powerful, as uterine contractions stimulate labor and work to bring the baby through the body and into the world. The sheer force of creation that rests in the uterus or womb can't be measured. If there is any doubt about your ability to transition from Maiden to Mother, if you are questioning your ability to surrender into and rise up to the challenge of birth, your womb can serve as the guiding force that reminds you that you are more than capable—that you are designed for this. "We have the universe within us, within our womb," explains Ulrike Remlein. "We have the elements of creation within our womb; that is why we can create babies. The power of the uterus is guiding you to find your strength from within. If you find that strength outside of yourself, you will be dependent on the outside world—that's not what you need when you give birth. You need to rely on yourself and on the bigger divine force working through you."

Acupuncture: A Tool for Late Pregnancy

In the weeks leading up to labor, regular visits to the acupuncturist can help prepare you for the big day. The practice "ripens the cervix" (as practitioners sometimes say) and can help move things along if you feel that you may go past the two-week window of your "due date" and end up being induced. Even if you get to that point but haven't seen an acupuncturist yet, it's not too late—a good practitioner will happily step up to treat you. Between appointments, try on some of the easiest (and the most fun) ways to get things moving: nipple stimulation, snuggling, laughter, and light touches from your partner (or yourself).

By beginning the process of trusting your body's ability, you're working against a lifetime of programming that tells women that we're not capable. As Rochelle Schieck explained, women are pushing against an unconscious conditioning that goes back to Adam and Eve—that her body is not trustworthy. You can play a significant role in unwinding that conditioning by focusing on your body's ability. When doubts creep in, see what happens if you simply believe in your biological capability, explains Lacey Haynes. "You could tell yourself, 'This is what my body is actually designed to do, so why can't I just get out of the way and let it happen? I can poop by myself. I can menstruate by myself. I can grow this child by myself. Isn't the natural next step to birth this child by myself?' Maybe that can be the thing we believe in more than believing things will go wrong."

You have a choice: You can be an active participant in your birth experience, claiming your sovereignty for the birth you desire, or cruise along on autopilot, allowing things to happen without expecting or asking for too much. To step up and actually be fully here for your birth, you will have to take responsibility rather than passing off all decision-making to someone in a white coat or blindly adhering to a set of universal guidelines that don't consider your unique experience. This is an active role that will ask you to release any inhibitions that may be holding you back. Lacey Haynes, ever the fierce advocate for connecting to your power, puts it this way: "If you can't realize yourself during birth, then you're going to be less powerful as a person in your life in general, because you weren't able to get pushed up against the edge of your discomfort and then actually rise to that."

By reading this book you're already bringing a level of awareness and intention to the entire baby-creation process. Educating yourself about how birth works, finding your ideal care providers, securing trusted people to lean on and share with, shaping your birth plan, understanding your rights as a birthing person, and taking a birth preparation class are all steps that help steep you in responsibility and intentionality. When you're informed, you may be able to see that you don't have to be induced or have another intervention; you can birth at your own pace and be that much closer to your ideal birth experience. An intentional birth, navigated with personal responsibility and clear intention, also paves the way for a more easeful post-partum period and smoother parenting as your baby grows. "We instantly see the positive impact on our lives. Right after birth, everything is easier," Lacey explains. "It's already a huge challenge to give birth and then to have this child who you have to nurse and take care of and who keeps you up at night, but you can slingshot yourself into a more successful transition if you've had a healthy birth that actually honored the

> You come into being through your mother and then you come into another level of being through your own life and yet another through having an intentional birth.
> —LACEY HAYNES

rhythm of your body." Lauren Curtain agrees. "With birth, so much changes, the more educated you are about it. Some women say, 'I'm just happy to do what my OB says, but that's how you end up with unnecessary intervention.' Being informed, understanding what the terminology means, can help you have an empowered and positive birth experience."

Birth can be magnificent, transcendent, enlightening, and empowering, but to have the birth of your dreams you first need to understand who you are and what's important to you. By moving through the five treasures, you embark on a journey of self-discovery that will help you understand your values. "I think that the more that you come into your own power in life and through your own self-development, birth then becomes just an extension of that," says Lacey Haynes. "And so then your birth reflects the way that you live your life."

Do Some Daydreaming

Allow yourself to daydream about your ultimate birth. "If you're planning to birth in a hospital, ask yourself, 'What does my dreamy birth look like?'" suggests Rochelle Schieck. "Ask yourself, 'What would it look like to be honored in this experience?'" Likewise, if you're planning to birth at home, can you encourage yourself to drop beyond the mere surface details and get to what it would look like to be honored in this experience?

Your vision of how you want to birth began the moment you chose your care provider(s), or even earlier if you found yourself dreaming of becoming a parent before you were even pregnant. You may have sketched out each step of your birth or you may have skipped over those details and headed directly to the part where your baby is nestled in your arms. If you haven't given a lot of thought to the birth experience that would help you feel safe, held, and empowered, now is a great time to start.

As you consider your ideal birth—understanding that birth is inherently mysterious, and at its core, unpredictable—it can be helpful to explore the roots feeding your beliefs about what you feel is possible for your birthing experience. Does the majority of what you believe to be true about birth come from what you

When we start to understand our values and then actually align our actions to our values, then our body becomes harmonized in a way that makes things like becoming pregnant and having babies so much more easeful and graceful, because all of the energy inside of our body is working in harmony with what we believe to be true. —LACEY HAYNES

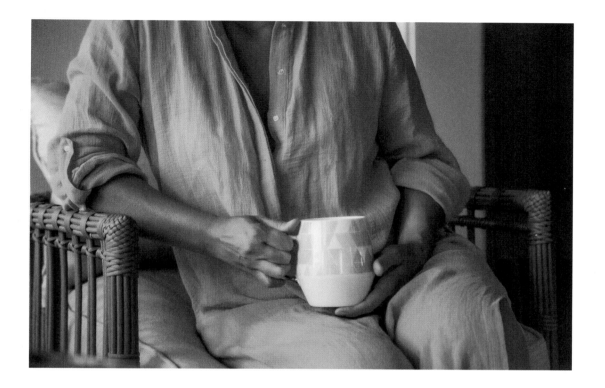

see in the media? Is your version of birth the screaming mom clenching the arm of her partner under glaring lights in a hospital room? Or does your concept of birth come from your family? Did your mom have a challenging time giving birth to you? How was your grandmother's birth experience(s)? Understanding your family history can help shape, or reshape, your idea of what birth can be. You can also create a new vision of what's possible for birth by using your time during pregnancy to saturate yourself with positive birth stories. Use your force field to take in only stories, images, and videos that leave a positive imprint. Be a fierce guard dog to what you let into your psyche. "I give my clients *good* birth stories. I tell them to flood their brains with good stories. It can optimize your birth," says Lauren. This doesn't mean you should shy away from the reality of the birthing process, but absorbing good stories and making small shifts when thinking about birth—like trading the word "contractions" for "surges" and "pain" for "sensation"—can create positive new pathways in your brain and alter your experience dramatically.

What's Your Birth Story? (Hint: Ask Your Mom)

If a woman has a fear about birth that keeps coming up as she gets closer to her birth time, it can get stronger—and there's a chance it can arise during labor. Sometimes as midwives, we don't hear about a fear the mother has until two weeks before birth—maybe she wasn't in touch with it before or she is embarrassed about what she's feeling. Often I'll have her ask her own mom what happened in labor. Without fail it was something. In fact, I typically say to *both* partners, if your mother is available to ask, try to bring it up and simply hear the first sentence that she shares about her birth experience. They'll get it in a nutshell. The details are not important; it's the emotion the mother has about it. From there, we can start to address the pregnant woman's fear with more awareness. —Davi Khalsa

As you settle into your vision of how you'd like your birth to unfold, fortifying yourself with tools that can support an empowered labor can help you shape the birth you're hoping to have. There are several popular birth preparation methodologies, and spending time with at least one of them can provide you with a foundation to lean into during the unpredictable waves of labor. It's worth doing some research to find the method that resonates with you. Many people find great benefit in HypnoBirthing™, The Bradley Method®, and Spinning Babies® (which can help babies turn in utero so they are ready for birth), and classes like San Francisco-based Yes to Birth!, which is based heavily on self-hypnosis. "I took Rachel Yellin's class (Yes to Birth!) and listened to the audio tracks that guide you to open your body and let go of fear," says new mom Rose Goldthwait. "It helps you enter into birth prepared to surrender to what is, without getting stuck in what could happen; it helps you go with what is happening in the moment, even if it feels huge. You continue to open and surrender." Attending courses like these might not only lift trepidation from your mind, it might—as several wise ones noted—make you feel quite giddy about what you're about to do.

> We so deeply believe that birth is broken, and we believe that women aren't capable of birth, and it's because we hear terrible stories.
>
> —LACEY HAYNES

Ask Questions!

If you have a question, ask it! Asking clear, direct questions throughout pregnancy can help you make empowered choices when you are in the throes of labor. If you feel shy, hesitant, or embarrassed to inquire about something, that's the sign that you absolutely need to ask. There are no stupid questions! Be a question-asking machine. Speak up during your birth preparation classes and at your prenatal appointments (and reach out between appointments if something is tugging at you). Ask other moms, care providers, even new acquaintances anything that's on your mind.

Do It Together

As you learned in Treasure Four, the Gift of Intimacy, you don't have to navigate pregnancy alone—or birth for that matter. As you prepare your mind and your heart for labor, factor in regular deep intimacy dives with your partner. This is especially important if your partner is going to be part of your birth support team—you are cultivating a sense of trust and safety that you will lean into when you go into labor. "The laboring person entrains with whomever they are sharing space with," explains Latham Thomas of Mama Glow. "During early labor it's necessary to create a safe space for the birthing person to move into the birth experience." Even though your partner will not be physically giving birth, they are stepping through the threshold into parenthood too, and this is a profound experience for them as well. They will be part of the container that creates the sacred space for your child to come through; by supporting your process and welcoming the newest member of your family, they are giving birth to a new version of themselves.

"When we are surrounded by the warmth, touch, and scent of our beloveds, we feel at ease. Before your doula or midwives arrive, or before you head to the hospital when labor is established—before anyone aside from the primary couple enters the space—the couple

> There is a connection between how you got pregnant and how you give birth. Birth and sex don't have to be so separate. Our society or culture has made them separate, but there is a capacity for birth being a sensual experience.
>
> —ROCHELLE SCHIECK

has a unique opportunity to create a container of safety," Latham says. "Turning off the highly stimulated neocortex—the thinking brain—allows the birthing person to enter an altered state using mind, body, and connection tools." This is your chance to revisit the space of touch you explored in the Gift of Intimacy. Your partner can offer you a massage, rubbing your feet and hands; you can dance, kiss, snuggle, and hold hands. Throughout pregnancy, and during the labor window, be sure to keep sensuality and physical intimacy and pleasure in the room. Staying connected in this way keeps the oxytocin pumping, supporting a smoother birth and keeping you and your partner in a warm cocoon of togetherness.

Consent Matters

After nine months of preparation, you are awake and aware, educated and informed, with a clear sense of who you are and what makes you feel safe and cared for. Your force field is up, allowing in only what feels right, and your intuition is honed and at the ready. You will be entering into your birth experience from a place of empowerment; this grounded sense of intention and responsibility will influence how your birth unfolds. Informed consent and shared decision-making have hopefully been with you throughout pregnancy, while you were asked to make choices about tests, procedures, or interventions, and they will remain with you throughout your labor journey too. Every care provider, including nurses, OBs, midwives, doulas, and anesthesiologists, must receive your consent before touching you or administering an intervention. Ideally, you will feel safe and protected by your care providers, trusting their expertise to help guide you to decisions that feel best for you and your baby, but ultimately you are your best advocate; the power lies within you. "No matter where or how you give birth, birth is your power play," says Khefri Riley. "Within medical systems, power is often taken away from birthing people, especially those from historically marginalized communities. We must not give our power away by allowing care providers to make unilateral medical decisions for us that aren't evidence based. I encourage parents to understand the benefits and risks of all procedures and to actively engage in

> I believe that if a woman isn't smiling and laughing in labor then someone isn't treating her well enough.
>
> —ROBIN LIM

THE SACRED TRINITY: MOTHER, BABY, PLACENTA

Part of a gentle landing for a new baby is honoring the stages after the physical birth: delayed cord clamping (you can request this from your care provider) and birthing the placenta. Delayed cord clamping means the baby's umbilical cord is not clamped and cut before the placenta has been safely born (and ideally, not for some time afterward), allowing extra time for the nourishing blood in the cord and placenta to flow to the baby. Delayed cord clamping can increase hemoglobin levels at birth and improve iron stores in the first several months of life, which is found to support positive developmental outcomes. Delayed cord clamping is the norm at Bali's Bumi Sehat. "We don't clamp and cut the umbilical cord for three hours," explains Robin Lim. "This protects the first embrace (where mother and baby remain skin to skin immediately after birth). It's everyone's human right to get that first embrace from your mother. We never take that away." Robin shares more wisdom about this profoundly important subject in her book, *Placenta, The Forgotten Chakra*. She writes, "At birth, it is important to be sure that the baby, placenta, mother, and family are truly ready for the umbilical cord to be cut. I believe that if the cord is to be severed at all, it is important to do this with reverence and pure intention, since once the baby-cord-placenta trinity is broken, it cannot be restored. . . . Take your time! Go slowly! There is no need to hurry or worry. Remember: Cutting the cord is not a rescue operation, though to see it done in hospitals you would think it is. It is indeed the rushing and the cutting that we need to rescue babies from."

collaborative, informed decision-making. Take classes and become familiar with current evidence-based practices. Let your provider know, 'I want shared decision-making at my birth.'"

Fully inhabiting your birth experience also means listening to what your body, and baby, are asking for, regardless of what anyone else is advising you to do. You may want to squat, walk, sing, dance, drape over your partner, eat soup with your best friend, or blast your hip-hop playlist. It's all good and all allowed. "The uterus is the most powerful muscle in the body, and at birth we are absolutely very powerful," shares Khefri. "So how convenient that modern obstetrics (which primarily is a white, male, heteronormative profession) puts us on our backs with our feet in stirrups taking our power! It's bonkers that a birthing person would believe they have to give their power over to anyone else. They should say, 'I hold the key to the primal intelligence of the universe within me! What do you mean I can't birth on my hands and knees?'"

When It Feels Like Too Much

You can be prepared, informed, fierce, and aware, and there will still inevitably be moments during birth that will feel overwhelming, even scary. This is expected. Giving birth is a huge initiatory experience that can bring up supreme vulnerability as you give way to a force that can feel bigger than you. When you meet places along the way that feel impossible to transcend—when you're too tired, too afraid, or in too much discomfort—don't forget that you have some serious tools in your toolbox now. You have your trusty force field, which can be used to keep out unwanted voices and energies from others, but also to keep unwanted thoughts out of your own mental landscape. (The practices in The Gift of Stillness can help you tame runaway thoughts.) By staying very present and surrendering to what is happening in the moment, you can avoid spiraling into whirlpools of treacherous thought. During her son's birth, Rochelle Schieck relied on a simple mantra to stay in the present moment and avoid tipping into a morass of "what ifs." "I would repeat, 'This is happening now . . . now this is happening.'" With your creative power in action, the worst-case scenario does not necessarily have to occur!

Access Your Animal Nature

Some women say, 'I'm going to die, I'm going to tear open, I can't do this.' It's such a real place for a lot of women. If they haven't worked on the mindset that you need when going into labor, then there's lots of surprises. If you have a mindset that this could be a long journey, or this is going to be hard, but I *can do* hard things, then anything that happens, you're OK. If you go into it with expectations, and those expectations are not met—it's taking longer than you thought or it's a little more intense than you thought—you could get really thrown. I encourage my birthing clients to connect to their animal nature, because animals don't have these blocks, they just birth their babies. —Haize Hawke

Ask the Ancestors for Help

Your support team is another tool there for you when you feel overwhelmed or afraid during birth. Lean on your people! Ask for help, tell them how you're feeling, and open yourself up to their tender, unwavering care. The value of choosing an experienced care team will shine here as your midwife or OB offers wise words and guidance to support you through the harder moments. But support is not limited to the physical realm. Many women say they felt connected to an ancient line of women who birthed before them—centuries and centuries of women who experienced the same thing. The circumstances surrounding their births may have been different than yours, but the challenge, and the gift, is the same. Feeling this ancient web of powerful creators can give you the fuel you need to make it over a hump that seems impossible to summit. You can tap into a general overarching, primal force that emanates from all the mothers that came before you, or you may choose to connect to some of your own ancestors.

You don't have to burn sage or get on your knees, unless that's how you feel like laboring, to access this ancestral support. "You just ask," explains Haize, who notes she has been attuned to her own ancestors' presence since she was young. "Ask for them to come and then they will come. I have found

> Some births aren't perfect, but when the baby comes out and gazes at the parents, the love is unshakable.
>
> —DAVI KHALSA

that the birth room is always crowded because the ancestors are always there, protecting and reminding the birthing person that they're not alone, that they have the resilience, energy, and power to do this." She shares how when a birthing person feels the love and support of their ancestors, the effect can be profound. "It gives the birther the courage to continue on—suddenly she has no fear and she has all the strength in the world to have a baby."

A New Birth for a New Baby

If this is your second or third baby (or more!) you may be working through trauma from your previous birth(s). It's natural to feel concerned that this birth will be like the births you've already had, but it's essential to remember that you are creating an entirely new being, and that you too are not the same person you were before. Be sure to discuss your birth history openly with your care provider with special attention on any specific worries you may have about the birth you're soon to have. Creating a new birth experience may be easier than you imagine.

Trusting in the Mystery of It All

There will be moments along your birthing journey where the most powerful thing you can do is nothing at all. And you are well prepared to do this: Confident in yourself, in your body, and in the support you've elicited, you can fully let go. Let go of the expectations of what this birth is "supposed" to be like; let go of any resistance to the fact that your body can and will bring this baby into the world. Let go of all the thinking. And there you will be: in your body and in the experience, accepting the unfolding of this birth as it is—whether or not it aligns perfectly with your plan. You are experiencing trust at the deepest level possible—trusting in the mystery. As you release your expectations about what your birth is supposed to look like and sink into knowing that your body is designed to bring your baby into the world, you open yourself up to experiencing the profound power of a body unfettered by the mind. When you get your head out of the equation, you accept the unfolding of your birth as it is, which may not be as you imagined.

Birth Matters for Baby Too

Though the onus has been on your maternal power until now—Shakti-filled creatrix that you are—part of that power involves creating a gentle landing for your baby. The interventions that you choose to have—or decline, like immediate cord cutting—and the space that you birth in, will influence what your baby's precious first moments will be like, an imprint that will be with them for the rest of their life. "At the moment of our death, we go through our life all the way back to our birth," shares Robin Lim. "And because the hearing of a baby is so acute at birth, we consider that what they hear when they're first born is going to be the last thing they remember of this life." This may sound intimidating, but it's also glorious. "What you say and sing in the beginning of life will set them on a path for the rest of their life. You can put a baby's feet on a really good path right at the beginning."

Consider the environment in which you will be birthing—not simply the tangible considerations, but the tone and feeling of the space as well. Even if the setting isn't your first choice, what can you do to make it feel warm and welcoming for your new baby? If you're giving birth in a hospital, bring your own lighting, music, blankets, and special objects that make you feel relaxed and happy—those feelings will be instantly transferred to your child. Talk to your care providers about how you would like the moments after birth to be handled so everybody understands your desires—even suggesting hushed tones for everyone in the room if you like. Remember, you have time to let your baby make the transition between worlds. Instead of being rushed to the next step of the process, can you let them experience skin-to-skin contact with you, with your and their smells, touches, and breaths all mingling together? This is sacred time! Thus it is wise to choose who will be in attendance with some discrimination. If you do want participants outside of your partnership, consider how beautiful it can be to have one or more people present who see this as a very sacred moment, and revere it as such. "As midwives, we're always singing as the babies are crowning," says Robin. "We all make sure that the moment of birth is acknowledged as a miracle, greeting the baby as a soul and not as a medical event."

Feed
Yourself
Well

The first time I learned about feeding a mother-to-be was when I was nineteen years old. My brother Hsuan and my tribe of cousins—Patty, Peter, Wendy, Joel, Tien, Phil, Chuan, An, and Brian—would regularly eat together at my Auntie Ou's home outside Oakland, California. I loved everything about those meals. The feeling of warmth and safety in her kitchen, with its three red oak trees standing guard outside (one for each of her children, Auntie Ou would sometimes say); the whisper of Buddhist chants and the fragrance of incense wafting in from Auntie's meditation room next door and mingling with the noise of children's chatter and aromatic cooking smells; and the reassuring, albeit bossy, presence of several matriarchs in the kitchen, offering a brusque but loving net of care while my own mother was in Maryland caring for her elderly mother.

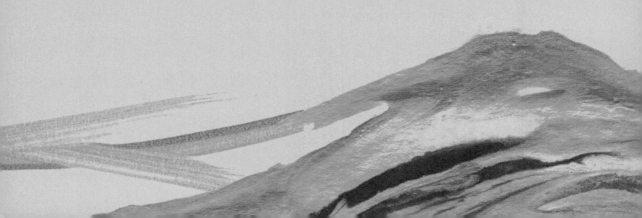

"Tree Aunt" as I sometimes called Auntie Ou, who is an acupuncturist known in the Bay Area for her fertility expertise, would hold court at those meals alongside Wendy's mom, Dr. Ju Chun Ou, and Patty and Peter's mom, Aunt Cathy. Of course, the star of these shows was the food itself. It was not fancy, but it was heavenly! These women took fresh market vegetables, simple cuts of meat, whole fish, and eggs, and transformed them through some kind of feminine alchemy—using a stripped-down collection of oil, black vinegar, salt, sugar, and white pepper for flavor—into the tastiest and most satisfying dishes we had all week. You couldn't sit at the table without getting into noisy chopstick fights for the best nuggets—like the gelatinous eyeballs of the catfish or the richest bit of bone marrow. When the braised greens and cabbage stew, the wood ear mushrooms, and the pork meatballs were set on the table for us to scoop from as we liked—shouts in Mandarin to get more rice for the elders and slurps of soup adding to the melee—each of us put the toppings in our bowls as we saw fit, guided by our appetites. We'd clean our bowls of every last grain of rice so as not to suffer the famed Chinese auntie glare.

But when Patty became pregnant, there was a subtle but perceptible shift in dynamics. Our eldest cousin got a promotion of sorts, elevated to a new position in our group. The aunties ordered us to make her comfortable, surrounding her with cushy pillows so she could nest into her spot. The younger ones were ordered to bring her nourishing broths and warm teas, and to set down our chopsticks so she got first dibs at the primo bits of meat. There was nothing precious about the scene—in fact, the more boisterous, the better, as our laughter and chatter kept Patty's spirits cheery and buoyed. Meanwhile, the elders buzzed around her with a steady murmur of directions to eat more of this and less of that—always noting her fluctuations in energy or mood and offering foods to support her where she was weak.

I hadn't thought of this scene much until my memories began to shape my MotherBees business. And I understood with a rush of raw emotion how the older women in the family were supporting Patty to step into her maternal power. They wanted her fortified and prepared, and nourishing meals were their primary tools. They barely spoke English and came from lines of Chinese medicine healers, so they most certainly didn't use the Western nutritional lingo we do today. But I see clearly now what they were doing. Through the smorgasbord of dishes they set out on that family table, they were letting her pick and choose from foods that would build her stores of critical nutrients—things like elongated fatty acids, found in silky custard eggs and sardines, that would grow her baby's brain and strengthen her own brain against postpartum depression; oodles of fat-soluble vitamins that helped her absorb minerals and use protein, and that would build her up to make breast milk later; and judicious amounts of red meat, along with red goji berries and jujube fruits, to ensure extra iron was available to help increase her volume of red blood cells, so more oxygen was available for her baby. And it went on! The arrays of ginger-braised greens, drizzled in sesame oil, pumped folate toward her fetus and kept her liver happy too, while the mushrooms boosted her immunity against germs she might otherwise fall prey to. Those famed fish heads we fought over? They were providing good amounts of iodine, so essential for her thyroid health and the subsequent balanced brain function of her child. Every so often, a "special energy" food would make an appearance in the mix, like fermented rice tonic to promote circulation and improve her levels of amniotic fluid, or delicate shavings of cooked snow fungus mushroom to support healthy bowels and counteract fatigue. But mainly what Patty was offered were the homey, simple foods we all ate regularly. What got ramped up was the deliberateness of the meals. The rest of us might be able to get by with skipping out on the protein occasionally or ditching the greens, but the mother-to-be couldn't do that.

To that end, these queens of the kitchen made it all extra yummy and hard to resist! Because they knew that a pregnant person's tolerance for eating can vary enormously. There are times when ravenous hunger hits, of course, and others when the desire to eat simply goes out the window—which can become a downward spiral of nausea and exhaustion if left unchecked for too long. Their firm directions to eat this and drink that were a tad overbearing, but they were love in action.

By the time I experienced my pregnancies, it was a little bittersweet that I was out on my own in Southern California, too far of a drive from Auntie Ou's Oakland Hills home to make it to family gatherings. Besides, most of the cousins had scattered by then. It wouldn't have been the same. Instead, the foundation of nourishment they'd laid into me over the years got expressed in new flavors entirely. My then-husband, raised on hearty English country fare, did his share of the kitchen prep. Succulent roast chicken, earthy potatoes smothered with local butter, and cauliflower mash enriched with farmhouse cream kept my body strong and my storehouses filled. I'd gone from East to West, exploring a new terrain. Where my cousin would have eaten warm rice congee for breakfast—a clean and neutral start to a day for a potentially queasy stomach—I enjoyed a modest cup of oatmeal, balanced with swirls of fat- and protein-rich nut butter, or a couple of hard-boiled eggs.

> Pull out all the stops when you are pregnant to ensure you eat well.
>
> —KAREN PAUL, *holistic nutritionist*

There was a gift in this distance, slightly sad as it may have been. It pushed me by necessity to be my own kitchen queen—to listen to the cues of my own body, rather than rely on others to say what they should be. I began gathering new teachings from the gurus on my path. When my brain felt foggy, I learned from a fishmonger that the fats from cold-water fish could give me an immediate aha, bringing me back. And when cravings for sugar pulled me off track, I learned from my beloved Davi that I actually needed more protein. Staying well fed during pregnancy wasn't always fun—and if you're pregnant as you read this, you might know exactly what I mean—but it helped me rev up a body sense that had been slowly growing since my teens. What did I need to eat when I was queasy, or tired, or anxious and ungrounded—or super jazzed to get stuff done? With so many different phases of pregnancy bringing different feelings, it was fertile practice ground for really listening in.

To be honest, I relish the freedom that came from not knowing too much information about pregnancy eating. Twenty years ago, and even fourteen years ago when I had my third child, Jude, expecting parents didn't have access to infinite and on-demand content like we do today. I was fortunate that, broadly speaking, I knew what to eat for all-around good health. (Auntie Ou and Co. had made sure of that!) And my instincts told me it didn't have to diverge too much from what I needed now. It never occurred to me to do endless study sessions in prenatal nutrition, as so many women feel they must do today! It was my own kind of approach: grounded in solid ingredients but guided by my intuition on what my body wanted me to feed it, day by day.

This has deeply informed how I cook for and with pregnant folks today. I believe that every person is going to have their own slightly different considerations for prenatal nutrition. As Auntie Ou likes to say, "Different body, different stomach, different baby." (My version of that is, "one size fits none"—I just don't like constrictive rules around food.) I'm a huge fan of working closely with your prenatal care provider to track how your nutrition is affecting your body. This includes asking questions about your blood sugar status and your iron and ferritin levels, keeping close tabs on your thyroid function throughout (even if your practitioner is trying to breeze past this often overlooked factor), and being curious about your vitamin D, magnesium, and B-12 vitamin levels too. (If your care provider isn't as interested as you are in this, don't be shy about stating why it matters to you.) Having one prenatal nutrition bible at hand, and reading it closely, is also incredibly helpful. From my MotherBees bookshelf, I often pull the books *Real Food for Pregnancy* by Lily Nichols or *The Nourishing Traditions Book of Baby & Childcare* by Sally Fallon Morell for pregnant friends and clients to read. My family's traditions teach that it's not wise to radically change your nutrition approach when pregnant, so for those following a less animal foods–rich diet, I might select Ibu Robin Lim's sweet and succinct book, *Eating for Two*, which "brings the midwife into the kitchen." One good primer can help you learn some solid foundations of how to get the right kinds and amounts of nutrients into your body for this tremendous period of growth and construction and help you in small but important ways to master the science of prenatal eating.

This then opens the space for what I hope to support you in here: the *art* of feeding your pregnant self well. I consider it the right-brain stuff to that left-brain effort. Because in my experience, ensuring you meet your protein needs, watch your carbohydrate intake, and include plenty of good fats, and choosing foods that give your body the array of micronutrients it requires, is actually fairly straightforward. You can use a scale or a cup measure for that part if you're so inclined, or you can eyeball that you have hit a good balance. Lots of experts will be happy to give you the numbers to aim for, and lists of minerals, fatty acids, and more.

But what is not so discussed is the less visible part of the equation: The attitude and atmosphere you create to care for your growing self through food. Do you have the heart to cook for yourself, day in and day out? Do you have the courage to ask others to cook for you when you feel you can't? Do the meals set down before you bring you comfort and solace—or are they just one more source of stress? Is the food you're eating making you feel warm and grounded and fed—or edgy, aggravated, or unsettled? This is the stuff that's hard to dig into in a brief prenatal visit and doesn't get social media eyeballs. But to me, it's the very heart of the matter.

I want to accompany you as you explore this very practical side of the golden pregnancy experience and offer you a hand to help you walk across its sometimes unsettled ground. Because let's be honest: What weirder phase in your eating career is there, really? On the one hand, eating during pregnancy is serious business—after all, the food you consume has to provide your body with fuel and fortification, plus all the building blocks for your baby and the reserves you will both draw from in postpartum. Yet this phase also asks you to hold your diet lightly and relax any viselike grip. Delight in eating one day can be followed by disdain or even downright disgust the next, all morphing into a kaleidoscopic blur. The types of foods you're drawn to can flip-flop, seemingly without rhyme or reason. The super-nutrient foods you thought you'd intake daily can feel utterly off-limits for weeks at a time. What other period of life serves up such a food paradox? You're asked to set up the best intentions in the world, then give them up, in part, to the great mystery, surrendering some of the control. Pregnancy eating is a microcosm of the whole pregnancy experience itself. Which means the attitude you take into it is as important as the ingredients themselves.

> Always remember you are eating for three considerations! Your own body's needs, those of your growing baby, and your future mothering reserves that you will draw on to feed your baby. Your reserves are your own personal treasure chest—don't let it get depleted; fill it up now.
>
> —DR. PADMA RAJU

When I contemplate the quieter influences on my cooking style, the ancestor who materializes in my mind is my maternal grandmother, who lived in Maryland. Not nearly as loud or recognized as the relatives on my paternal line, Granny Po-Po was the granddaughter-in-law of the renowned herbalist Dr. Huang, and she had wanted to study Western medicine but was thwarted by war. She was underestimated for her soft-spoken ways, and blind in one eye. I see now how she quietly poured generations of healing wisdom into her food. As a kid, I loved being at Granny's elbow as she wrapped sticky rice in lotus leaves, then tied the bundles up with string to place in the steamer. She had lived through many challenges, and the kitchen was a place of solace. From her I picked up how the everyday rituals of making simple food can be infused with more than words can say.

If I were cooking at your side during your months of pregnancy, I'd want you to feel your kitchen as a place where you can sink into yourself for a spell of time, getting out of your head and into your body—a place where you feel calm and connected, and the opposite of flustered or stressed. I'd want you to feel like you've already done more than enough just by showing up, and that it honestly doesn't matter if you have the perfect pantry already organized—because we can improvise together, if the bare bones of it are good. The very simplest of foods will often satiate and suffice, even if they don't feel especially groundbreaking or new. In fact, I'd want you to feel a sense of reassurance from the fact that none of this is new! When I get my hands on my favorite ingredients, like knobs of ginger or handfuls of spring greens, it reminds me that other women have done this before me, many times over. It lifts intimidation out of cooking and makes me feel comforted and not alone. My grandmother's hands did the same thing my aunts' hands did and eventually, mine and my cousins' too. As wild as this may seem now if your days are packed with demands, I'd love you to feel, somewhere in yourself, that your kitchen is a place you return to in order to get settled, not a place to run away from with angst or dread.

And most importantly, I'd want you to experience what it's like to receive a meal that feeds you deeply. I'd want you to sit down with relief, take a moment to exhale, and notice what washes over you when nourishing food is set before you. Someone has noticed you're hungry, and the food is ready. Could you feel the glow of contentment beginning to radiate, from your belly outward, anticipating the first bite or sip? For me, that handover moment is what cooking for and with mothers is all about. And it can exist for you whether you are your own chef or are being fed by another.

Deliberate and Kind

MAKING EATING WELL YOUR PRIORITY

If you feel you've launched into pregnancy with an uncertain relationship to food, you are far from alone. So many people have been in a rocky relationship with their diet before they conceive a child, fretting about it or even fighting with it for years. For others, good nutrition is more like an on-again off-again thing. (Who hasn't promised themselves, *I'll cook that lentil-vegetable soup tomorrow, really I will!*). Other times (oftentimes, in fact) the resistance to prepping wholesome food consistently runs a little deeper than that; it's coming from a low sense of enoughness, the sense we haven't done enough yet today, haven't achieved enough yet, to claim the time slot for prepping and eating something satisfying. If you're already a mother, you might know this as the "scavenge my kid's leftovers for dinner" scenario; or maybe it's "I'm so over trying to figure it out, I'll just have a glass of wine and go to bed."

Make a pledge
to eat right,
even if in the
beginning you
don't like it!

—DR. DANMEI HU,
acupuncturist

Until all of a sudden you are pregnant, and the force of sheer biology makes those old approaches obsolete. With all that is getting constructed in there, skimming by on a wish and prayer, or chronically shortchanging yourself around eating simply cannot work anymore. Just think of what is occurring! Not only is a human being constructed (six to nine pounds of him or her, most typically), but so is a whole new organ of your own— your placenta, a whopping pound and a half in weight on average. Plus there's a curling, robust umbilical cord, significant new volumes of blood, and a small ocean of amniotic fluid, not to mention the tissue and fluid that makes your uterus expand exponentially. And your breasts get bigger too. This is a very real construction project, and the materials do not come from thin air. They come from what you eat (and what you have been eating for the months prior—hence the importance of preconception eating). Though I'm far from a math whiz, if you add up exactly what is growing in a pregnant person, the scope of this hits home. You're adding at least twenty-five to thirty pounds of baby-related body matter alone. I can't help but envision all the cells of an expecting mother doing a nine-and-a-half month long refrain: "Honey, listen up, I'm building a kid; I'm fortifying you to give birth;

I'm making a placenta and growing an umbilical cord; I'm stockpiling nutrients for breast milk, while also powering all your normal activities too. So here's my order—ample protein and plenty of iron, really good fats every day, hydration that hits the spot, and the full array of vitamins and minerals like you've never consumed them before. And by the way, the only way I can get this stuff is from you!" If eating ever was an afterthought, it can't be that any longer. Your pregnant body will ask nourishment to become your first consideration, not your last.

Ask any person who's been pregnant and they likely would agree that it's a phase in which everything is amplified, from surges of hunger so strong you want to flag down the nearest hipster food truck to the strange or infuriating experience of days (or weeks) in which eating anything at all seems like a cruel joke. Or you may experience extremes of indigestion, new depths of spaciness, or moments of fatigue so profound you can't imagine how you ever stayed up past 8:30 p.m. before. And at the center of many of these sensations is what you have or have not consumed. Your diet can help you ride through this physical metamorphosis smoothly when it's right for you, or it can contribute to a rodeo ride when it's not.

The wise ones who buzz around the MotherBees hive have taught me how many common pregnancy concerns are often a result of poor nutrition, and not the consequence of bad luck or faulty genes. By the same token, they can often resolve themselves with good nourishment and lifestyle changes. Nausea, a common early pregnancy sensation caused primarily by hormone changes, gets exacerbated from not eating and letting blood sugar drop too low (and is made worse, according to some experts, by shirking protein). Morning sickness can be worse when magnesium stores haven't built up for several months in advance. The blood sugar dysregulation that can lead to gestational diabetes is brought on by a high-carbohydrate diet laden with sugars and refined grains. Many have felt the fatigue or even full-blown anemia that can come as naturally increasing blood volume is not met with corresponding increases in iron levels. Even high blood pressure, hypertension, and preeclampsia, as well as hypothyroidism, are considered by many to be conditions brought on by nutrient deficiency. Wise one Karen Paul, a holistic nutritionist and friend in Hawaii who often counsels women on fertility and pregnancy, shared with me how the work of the pioneering 1960s doctor Tom Brewer was some of the first to link malnourishment to all these conditions, with a distinct emphasis on protein lack.

Not surprisingly, the amplification effect plays out just as much in your mental and emotional well-being. Consider how even in a non-pregnant state, running out of fuel creates system-wide stress. Factor in the demands of pregnancy, and the effect of being under-resourced gets turbocharged. As wise one Damian Hagglund says, the quickest way for anxiety to take hold during pregnancy is forgetting to eat and drink and letting your gas tank hit "empty." (And when stress hits, it's all too easy to turn to comfort foods high in sugar or processed ingredients that tax the body more.) The good news is that, conversely, when you do stay nourished and practice anticipating and avoiding those running-on-fumes moments by having good food on hand (or better yet, loved ones helping you anticipate it), you lay in powerful prevention against the ravages of physical and mental stress, for yourself and your baby.

In a way, even with all the up and down sensations that can come with pregnancy eating, your body is giving you a gift. When you are pregnant, it will pretty much demand you feed it what it needs to function, no holds barred. If in the past you were able to override those needs—fueled by sheer willpower or coffee and energy drinks—now, the game is up. And where it might be possible to postpone some of the other basic elements of personal care, like meditating or getting sunlight on your skin, eating can't be postponed for long. You tend to do it several times a day.

In the best-case scenario, your relationship with eating has gotten some tending and, if needed, healing in your preconception months or years (something my co-writers and I outlined in *Awakening Fertility*), and it's become easier to see healthful eating as the mothering ally that it is. One of the focuses of *Awakening Fertility* is avoiding today's norm of entering pregnancy in an already depleted state. Poor quality food stripped of its nutritional value, stress, compromised gut health, and the depleting effects of hormonal birth control are just four of the reasons for this state of lack. In that book, we shared how the months (or years) before conception are the ideal time to turn that around, especially because it sets you up strongly if eating well is a challenge in the first trimester. If you haven't had that prep time, however, you are far from alone. The time to layer in fortification and gains is now! And what an opportunity it is—a forty-week experience in squeezing the most goodness out of your food.

WHY GOOD FOOD MATTERS

Perhaps the most persuasive argument for putting some elbow grease into eating well while pregnant is this: We are learning how the nutrients in our foods have decreased dramatically in the last hundred years. At the heart of the problem are soils saturated with life-killing biocides and stripped of minerals as a consequence of modern farming methods, and processed foods that have left nature's nutrients on the factory floor. Our bodies' biological needs, however, have not decreased dramatically! Most especially when it comes to creating a new human and recovering from the process ourselves. A baby in utero, and its ally, your placenta, will take whatever it needs from its mother's bones, tissues, teeth, and even brain tissue to develop as best it can, literally pulling nutrients from her own stores; if those nutrients aren't there in sufficient quantity in this time, baby's lifelong health can be affected. Furthermore, as the ancestral traditions teach, mom's ability to recover, rebuild, and reproduce again can be highly compromised from lack of nutrients before and during each pregnancy. A long-lasting state of depletion, and even postpartum depression, can be hard to ward off when the materials the body and brain require to function have been (literally!) sucked away. Luckily, if you take a keen interest in your ingredients, prepping as many meals and snacks as possible from whole foods and choosing ingredients packed with nutrition (also known as nutrient-dense foods), you are in a much better position to avoid these things. A well-chosen prenatal supplement can most certainly play its part in this project, and I always recommend asking your trusted care providers for brands of the highest quality. A prenatal vitamin is like an insurance policy, backing you up by helping fill the nutrition gaps that invariably occur as a fact of modern life. Just don't rely on it to be your foundation. The credo "You can't out-supplement a poor diet" rings true in pregnancy as in all phases of life.

The Seven Guidelines

Have you noticed how many food taboos pop up the minute you discover you're pregnant? Don't let any dirt remain on those farmers' market carrots (a bacterial risk), no soft cheese (many say ditto), be wary of sushi (in case it has parasites), or go cold turkey on caffeine (in case it increases miscarriage risk). Perhaps, due to certain health conditions you're working with, entire categories of macronutrients or food groups are on the "no" list (like highly refined carbohydrates if you are a candidate for gestational diabetes, or gluten if you have gluten sensitivity or autoimmune thyroid conditions). These are valid considerations and, like any basic safety measures, are important to heed. But I've noticed how the focus on what *not* to eat can, if we're not careful, lead to a kind of stultifying confusion around what to cook, or a frozen kind of inaction, or even a lurking dread that danger awaits with every bite.

It's so very important to not feel shut down around food in this all-important time! In order to open it up, I want to offer you a different perspective, one that focuses primarily on all that you *can* eat, and then helps you use food as a way to stay connected to, and deeply care for, yourself.

Chances are if you're reading this book—a pregnancy book with food on the cover!—you've already put some thought into prenatal nutrition. Perhaps you have already picked a team, so to speak, and are drawn to the nutrient-dense "sacred foods" of the Weston A. Price approach, or the colorful Mediterranean diet espoused by mentors like our friend Dr. Aviva Romm, or even an Ayurvedic or Chinese medicine-inspired diet for pregnancy. Perhaps you simply are hoping to eat as "clean" as you can—low in chemicals and high in whole foods. As my cowriters and I put together this chapter, we each had our own (sometimes fierce) allegiances to the dietary approaches we felt served our bodies, and our babies, best. Yet we also made a fascinating discovery as we interviewed the wise ones working in the field. The people who actually take care of pregnant women, day in, day out, speak in softer and more allowing terms around diet than many of the books and blogs and online mama groups do! They're really in it, they've seen it all, and the reality is that getting nourishment over the nine-plus months of being pregnant is rarely a textbook situation.

Seven precepts for a solid nutritional foundation stood out in all our conversations; simple and to the point, they align beautifully with how I cook, both at home for my children and myself, and in the MotherBees kitchen for moms. If you keep these guidelines within reach, I feel confident you will be on very sure footing. I think of them as seven brushstrokes—gestures that put the outline of a picture on the canvas, but let you fill in the colors, textures, and nuances in a thousand different ways to suit your style.

1

Eat Real Food

Eat whole foods in their original, untampered states as much as you can, and steer clear of packaged, processed foods as much as your circumstance makes possible. Go light on store/deli-made and take-out meals if you can. Try to source as many meals, snacks, and beverages from the ingredients in your fridge or pantry. (The herbal teas included in the Recipes section can be enjoyed at room temp or warm.) This is your number-one way to have the most control over quality. From a traditional Ayurvedic perspective, fresh foods from nature are full of prana, the subtle life force of the universe, and they help build the quality of *ojas*, which is the biochemistry of well-being, longevity, and bliss for both mother and child. Fresh vegetables and fruits, freshly prepared legumes, quality dairy, blanched (skinned) almonds, coconut, and dates are famously known as sattvic foods, increasing the qualities of purity and clarity as they nourish deeply. In speaking to our wise ones, we heard many times how these fresh, simple foods popping with vitality should be prepared simply during pregnancy, without complex flourishes and over-the-top flavors. Let the vibrancy of the food really sing! Of course, you're going to likely consume something that comes in a box or package as part of even a whole-foods

> Always we have fewer spices, fewer garnishes on the food—it's about more sattvic food that's easily digestible, and easily assimilated during pregnancy.
>
> —DR. PADMA RAJU

approach. If a food or drink item comes in a package, at least do this: take three seconds to flip it over and read the ingredients. What nutrients are they offering you? What additives (sugars in particular) have been smuggled in?

2

Eat Protein with Every Meal or Snack

Protein is your biggest baby building block, and you need it, in generous amounts, to get the job done. Gestation, labor, postpartum recovery, breastfeeding—each phase has its protein demands, so don't skip out! It is also satiating and filling, and when we get enough, we don't crave sugar-spiking carbs as much. When I read Lily Nichols's brilliant book *Real Food for Pregnancy* and learned how adequate protein helps regulate blood pressure during pregnancy, thanks to the amino acid glycine that is found in the gelatin- and collagen-rich connective tissues, skin, and bones of animal foods, and that glycine also protects against the oxidative stress that is a hallmark of preeclampsia, I had an aha moment—no wonder my Chinese matriarchs pushed the pork-feet broth, slow-cooked meat stews, and crispy cracklings toward the pregnant eater so often! (Robin Lim also taught me how eating adequate protein when pregnant wards off restless, tossing-and-turning nights.) Chances are you already know how many options exist for protein sources, both animal and plant-based. Know that when you choose a fully grass-fed or pasture-raised animal sourced protein (meat, eggs, and dairy), you not only get a complete protein, you may be getting bigger doses of essential fatty acids and micronutrients too, due to the nutrient-dense foods and forage the livestock ate. (Much of these are in the fats, which is why traditional diets did not favor "lean protein" as some dieticians do today!) Eggs, for their part, deliver affordable protein with baby brain–building choline, critical B vitamins, and

Protein Sources

Beef, lamb, chicken, pork, buffalo, liver and organ meats, chicken and turkey, bone broth, sardines and other fish low on the food chain, wild salmon, yogurt, eggs, cheese, legumes/beans (lentils, mung beans, garbanzo, black, kidney, white, etc.), quinoa, spirulina, pumpkin and hemp seeds, gelatin/collagen powders, protein powders (grass-fed whey, organic plant protein including pea protein and pumpkin seed), nuts and nut butters in moderation—almond, peanut, walnut, cashew.

A Note on Dairy

Dairy foods can be a wonderful addition to pregnancy eating for their protein, good fats, calcium, and, when fermented, their gut biome-boosting probiotics. Bodies respond differently to dairy foods, however. Many find that pasteurized cow dairy makes them feel congested or mucus-y (or "damp" and sluggish in the Chinese medicine vernacular—the opposite of the warm, cozy temperature your pregnant body may want). Others don't notice that at all. It's interesting that traditions that advocate daily milk in pregnancy, such as Ayurveda, typically use milk from older breeds of cattle that only produce the A2 dairy protein. In the US and Europe, most cow milk sold in stores comes from hybrid cattle that produce a mix of A1 and A2 proteins, making the milk harder to digest and more likely to have an inflammatory/ mucus-y effect. Goat milk is naturally A2 and a great option to try for easier digestion; genuine A2 cow milk is getting easier to source as well. One note: Please ensure dairy products are full fat, and free of added sugar. Many people love using Greek yogurt at this time as it is higher in protein than other kinds—and it tends to have no flavorings or sweeteners added. I suggest noticing how dairy products make you feel and experiment with sources if you like. It's always recommended to drink milk warm or hot, never cold; yogurt or kefir can also be enjoyed closer to room temperature if you like. See the recipe for Warming Cardamom Rose Milk on page 235 for one way to enjoy it. Please note: Dairy foods can inhibit the absorption of iron, so eat them separately from your Blood-building foods (see page 155).

vitamin A (absolutely vital for baby's development), and the brain-building fatty acid DHA. Bone broth, in addition to delivering all-important glycine, is replete with desperately needed minerals like calcium and magnesium. In the super-protein category come organ meats like liver, a renowned nutritional powerhouse that fills your stores of vitamin A, vitamin B12, and iron in the form that will be especially well utilized by your body. And don't forget fish, a source not only of protein but those ultra-essential omega-3 fatty acids, as well as trace minerals like selenium that help protect you from accumulating mercury. Small fish like sardines, herring, anchovies, as well as salmon are among the safest bets. (Note, in Chinese tradition, the crustaceans like crabs, shrimp, and prawns are considered overly chilling for this phase of life.) Of course, plant-based sources of protein are also very important to include. They'll add so much diversity to your plate. Lentils, mung beans, soybeans, and garbanzos (think hummus!), pumpkin and hemp seeds, quinoa, nuts and nut butters (not forgetting pistachios, a complete protein), and even the blue-green algae spirulina are some of the other options for meeting this essential need. Where eating a diet with animal foods will give you the full array of amino acids needed (the building blocks of protein), strict vegetarians must pay special attention to combining foods well to get the complete array of amino acids the body needs, including that all-important glycine. One piece of advice repeated by almost every care provider I have spoken with: Vegan mothers need significant special support to avoid deep depletion, especially in their second or later pregnancies; for some, adding in select animal products, with reverence, during the childbearing and breastfeeding year will be a wise option, even if they choose to return to their plant-only diet later.

3

Fill Your Plate with an Abundance of Vegetables

Eat vegetables of all colors and textures—leafy, crunchy, and starchy. Cooked vegetables are my preference over raw for their ease of digestion and assimilation. Use vegetables to crowd out high-carbohydrate staples that tend to get supersized on Western plates (bread, pasta, and other refined grain-based products). These foods often have a high glycemic index and can contribute to dysregulated blood sugars, especially during pregnancy. (A tip is to ensure the carbohydrate-dense foods like whole grains and starchy vegetables occupy only a small space on the plate, with leafy/crunchy vegetables and protein taking up most of it.) Enjoying oodles of veggies, ideally cooked or drizzled with some healthy fat on them, is not just for the obvious vitamin and mineral fix (like vitamin C, folate, calcium, and magnesium, the latter three all found in leafy greens). It's also for the all-important fiber, which in addition to stabilizing blood sugar and making you feel full, crucially feeds the health-giving bacteria colonizing your gut. Your gut microbiome may be out of sight but it should be far from out of mind. When it is balanced and thriving, it supports your immunity, a balanced brain state and mood, and healthy, regular elimination among many other things. When your bowel movements are full of

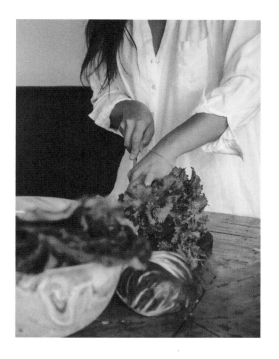

healthy bacteria, this does spill over, so to speak, to help colonize your vaginal microbiome—which will start to build your baby's health-giving microbiome after birth. I love including vegetables with high prebiotic value. ("Prebiotic" means they feed the probiotic organisms living in your gut.) These include radicchio, asparagus, artichoke, jicama, leeks, onions, palm hearts, and also apples. (Try the Rujak recipe on page 225 using jicama and apple!) In addition, small condiment portions of fermented veggies (like sauerkraut, kimchi, lacto-fermented relishes, and pickles) will help your biome flourish, which boosts another pregnancy superpower: your gut sense. (As co-writer Amely likes to remind me, the bacteria in our gut biome communicate information about our environment directly to our brains—a recently understood scientific phenomenon!) Don't forget, you can also feed your microbiome with fermented dairy products (yogurt, kefir, and the like) and drinks like beet kvass, water or fruit kefir, and kombucha in moderation. (Most kombucha has some caffeine in it from the tea it's brewed from, and it can have significant sugar content.)

4

Embrace Good Fats

This is not the time to eat low-fat. I suggest having an array of traditional real-food fats: butter, ghee (aka clarified butter), coconut oil, avocado oil, and good quality (pasture-raised) lard or tallow, and using unheated or only mildly heated virgin olive oil as a drizzling agent. Please don't cook with so-called "vegetable oils," which are processed oils sourced in industrial seeds or soybeans, not vegetables!

Easily rancidified and typically inflammatory, they are not your friends, and many experts feel they are as hazardous as sugar to our health. (This is another reason to avoid processed foods and to be careful about eating deli-prepared meals, which are typically laden with vegetable oils such as canola and soybean oil.) I'd also be cautious about nut oils and toasted seed oils—if used, keep in a cool, dark space and use quickly to avoid rancidity. When you pick bright yellow, grass-fed butter or golden ghee, or add lush cream from a great source to a dish, you get a big serving of important fat-soluble vitamins, especially vitamin K2, which is pivotal in your baby's formation and genetic expression.

5

Reduce Your Sugar Intake Significantly

Or (sorry to say it) reduce it almost completely. This includes honey, agave, and maple syrup too—keep them in small amounts! Given that so many people today enter pregnancy in an already slightly compromised state (with blood sugar levels in the prediabetic range, according to many experts) we don't have the wiggle room to play fast and hard with sugar. Fruits can satiate the desire for sweets— my aunties suggest having moderate portions of juicy fruit in the morning to hydrate and nourish, and using fruits in cooked dishes, as you will find in both savory and sweet recipes that follow. (I even like finding the naturally sweet taste in beans, which Asian kitchens sometimes turn into treats.) When a true sugar yearning calls, a small amount of dark chocolate (organic and 70 percent cacao) twice a week is what my dear Davi would allow. I have included some low-sugar treats starting on page 224. (At MotherBees, we are also fans of an occasional small portion of warm custard, like the recipe we shared in *The First Forty Days*, which is essentially rich ice cream before it is frozen, to avoid the dreaded maternal chill.) Today, it has become easier than ever to live sugar smart, because so many new products exist that give a sweet taste without sugar or nasty artificial sweeteners. We often use Swerve sweetener in lieu of sugar, or SunRoot liquid sweetener, which is packed with prebiotic inulin for good measure. And if you are truly hankering for candy? Seek out the new zero-sugar candies like SmartSweets, also made with prebiotic sweetening agents!

The Traditional Perspective

A grandmother's kitchen will have a true smorgasbord of ingredients when cooking for a mother-to-be. One group of foods in the Chinese tradition is the Blood-building foods, which loosely stated are what we in the West could consider foods rich in iron (though that doesn't quite capture the full scope of how these foods help build your Blood). Beef, beef bone broth, beets, eggs, dark leafy greens, blackstrap molasses in moderation, liver, dark berries, seaweed (especially dulse), almonds, pistachios, dates, sweet potatoes (purple color), black sesame seeds, and mushrooms are all considered Blood-building. Another, lesser known category of pregnancy foods are "reinforcement foods," which are prized for their ability to help the development of baby's organs in the first and second trimester. Perhaps surprisingly, they are not all "nutrient-dense" in feel. They include spring cabbage, spinach, sesame, white fungus, coconut, and beans, including black beans. The recipes that follow offer creative ways to enjoy some of these foods—even white fungus, which, odd as it may sound, is simply a mushroom. All told, there's a cornucopia of foods to enjoy in this special time—so have fun and have at it!

6

Stay Hydrated

You are helping build your increasing blood volume and create amniotic fluid for your baby to float in. A good top end to aim for is about eight to ten 8-ounce (237 ml) cups of filtered water per day—maybe a little more in summer, less in winter. Drinking filtered water hot or warm (or room temperature, but never cold) is ideal; sipping on hot water is a time-tested technique for grounding the vata that can cause aggravation when in excess. Fresh vegetables and fruits also add to your hydration, as do soups, broths, and stews. Staying well hydrated will serve you during labor too, helping keep contractions moving along. To support optimal hydration, be sure that your whole-foods diet includes sprinklings of quality salt. (I like to use good sea salt, with iodine added.) Sodium helps keep the balance of fluids in the body regulated; shirking salt too much actually throws this balance off.

7

And Remember to Eat as Kindly as You Can

Pregnancy can be one of the most heartopening times of your life, when you feel most compassionate and, sometimes, the most connected to nature and the cycles of life. This is a wonderful time to give the sources of your food your best attention; firstly, do your very best to use organic dairy, eggs, grains, and legumes, and go organic for as many of the vegetables and fruits as you can (especially the pesticide-heavy "Dirty Dozen" vegetables and fruits listed on ewg.org). The effects of pesticides on the baby in utero are profound and include affecting their hormones and cognitive development. It is especially important to try your very best to avoid grains and legumes that have been grown or treated with the notorious herbicide glyphosate—think conventional wheat, corn, and soy in particular. Organic products will by definition be free of this dangerous chemical, and so will non-GMO products, though non-GMO products will likely have been sprayed with other biocides instead. There's just too much risk to your baby's health and development to ignore this inconvenient truth. When it comes to meats and fish, it

You Don't Necessarily Have to Supersize Your Plate While You're Pregnant!

Caloric requirements gradually increase, mainly starting in the second trimester, but not as much as you might think. A 15 to 20 percent higher caloric intake is generally recognized as reasonable, depending on your metabolism and activity level. If, like me, you have never counted a calorie in your life, you will likely do great by consuming enough food, including healthy snacks, to satiate your hunger, without going past that point. This can be a pretty good guide when your diet comprises primarily whole (unprocessed) foods, keeps refined carbohydrates and sugars low, and includes plenty of protein, good fats, and diversity. (Make those plates and bowls full of color!) I would rather you focus on increasing the quality of food as much as possible, upping the micronutrient supply as best you can, and let your appetite regulate quantity. As always, work closely with your care provider for individualized support around healthy weight gain.

Golden Ghee

Of all the foods consumed during this "golden time," one of the most treasured is ghee, or clarified butter (which means the milk proteins are separated out, leaving only the fat). Long considered an elixir of life in India, where it's often recommended to take at least one spoonful daily during pregnancy to help baby's immunity and vitality, a daily dose of ghee will aid your digestion and elimination, calm your nerves, and help with sound sleep. Use it to sauté your proteins or vegetables, stir it into warm drinks, spread it on cooked vegetables, stir it into grains, or spread it on small amounts of toast. Since the proteins are removed, this can typically be enjoyed by those who are dairy sensitive. (It's possible to find certified protein-free ghee if you are very sensitive.) Ghee is also easy, and very satisfying, to make yourself!

is preferable to find fully grass-fed and pasture-raised meat from providers known for high standards, which will not only be free of chemical inputs but may have better nutritional profiles. That can feel out of reach to some—and the challenge is real, financially. But it can be made more doable by braising/slow cooking cheaper cuts of meat, using bones for broth, or going in on bulk orders of frozen meat with friends. Eating meat becomes a whole different experience when you find purveyors who treat animals with terrific welfare and practice regenerative land management (like our friends at Georgia's White Oak Pastures, or the many other regional providers found through eatwild.com). When it comes to seafood, the dilemma is mind-boggling these days. Once you know about the damage that industrialized fishing is causing, you can feel frozen, unsure whether to eat any at all. But fish and seafood contain so many important nutrients for you and your baby, I feel the best path forward is to educate yourself as best you can at this time about overfishing and damaging practices, make thoughtful choices, and get the nutrients in now, even if your conscience has you pull back from fish consumption in post-baby years.

The stakes are high when pregnant; yet it's also wise to keep things in perspective. If you cook with these seven guidelines in mind and use ingredients that come from the best sources you can access or afford, you are laying down a firm foundation. You can up the ante from there, of course: dialing up the nutrient

STAR PREGNANCY FOODS

Explore a few ingredients you may not normally enjoy.

Fish eggs, also known as roe, caviar, or ikra or ikura: This is quite possibly the crème de la crème of fertility and pregnancy foods (and considered a powerhouse "first food" for babies too!) It's chockablock with iodine, zinc, DHA, and fat soluble vitamins, as well as healthy cholesterol. Try it if your brain feels foggy or unsettled! Salty and crunchy-soft in the mouth, it's ideal to get the best quality you can get—Alaskan sourced wild salmon eggs are good. Beware of imported "caviar" that may be dyed black or treated with chemicals. Spread on crackers with cream cheese, top slices of hard boiled eggs, or get creative!

Blanched almonds are considered to be ojas-building foods in Ayurveda; they also have good protein and fat and may help settle a queasy tummy. Dr. Padma Raju has her pregnant clients eat six to eight of them every morning to start the day strong. A quick YouTube search will show you how to easily blanch almonds (the skins are considered irritating).

Ginger can be a true pregnancy supporter, especially in battling morning sickness. When consumed in moderation, it may help ease nausea while supporting circulation, helping to increase warmth in the body. Try it in the Millet Ginger Congee (page 182) or the Asian Pear Ginger Tea (page 233).

Jujubes are the MotherBees star fruit. Crunch them fresh like small apples or use the air dried version for soups and teas. The ruby red fruit is high in fiber, vitamin C, and antioxidants, and is used in Chinese medicine to support digestion, sleep, and anti-aging. We love them in Warming Jujube Tea (page 231) and Chicken Ginger Rice Soup (page 186).

Walnuts nourish kidney yang (which supports the warming hormone progesterone), provide good fat and protein, and can treat low back pain and constipation. Snack on them throughout the day or try them in Cardamom Breakfast Bowl (page 214) or sprinkled on Cacao Chia Pudding (page 226). Be sure to keep them refrigerated to prevent rancidity.

density with primo pregnancy foods. But if more often than not you are loosely following these guidelines, rest assured you are doing great! I believe that junk thoughts are as bad as junk foods—and if you hold yourself to outrageous standards of perfection, it is easy to self-sabotage. One of the best things you can consume is love for all that you are pulling off, not loathing for all you are not.

Unfolding into Your Knowing

THE GOLDEN OPPORTUNITY OF PREGNANCY EATING

Food is turned into nourishment by a process that involves physical digestion, yes, but also involves your mind (with your state of relative stress or ease being a big factor in how well you digest and absorb nutrients), your senses (they steer you toward food you feel inspired to cook and eat), and your heart (because self-love and the ability to receive factor into this equally too). In Treasure One, I shared the legacy of pampering the pregnant person, held in a net of care. I'd love for that feeling to infuse, at least some of the time, into your experience of eating your daily meals. As it turns out, the four golden guidelines shared by our wise ones about pregnancy at large apply beautifully in the kitchen.

1

Be Gentle with Yourself

Take nutrition seriously, yet treat yourself gently. Do your best to eat consistently, with some grace for any moments when you just can't. Especially in the early phases, as your body is adjusting to pregnancy, all kinds of sensations—dizziness, tiredness (or downright exhaustion), poor focus, and the oft-mentioned spectrum of queasiness (from mild to pronounced)—might throw a wrench in your nutritional plans. Paradoxical as it may seem, the more you can take in balanced, protein-rich meals, the better you may feel. Neutral and warming is the way to go—think simple chicken soup, or if that's too much for you, sip Golden Chicken Ginger Broth (page 185), lightly salted. If there are moments you can't stand to eat at all, well, eat when you can. "Try to eat regularly and keep your blood sugar stable," says Lauren Curtain. "This supports your Stomach and Spleen, which produces Blood and chi, so you feel more energy." (If nausea and vomiting become severe, please alert your prenatal care provider.)

Likewise, the way meals look can change a lot over your forty-ish weeks. Be open to that fluctuation. Meal size and/or frequency may well change from regular programing. In the first trimester especially, small bites throughout the day (or even by your bedside at night) may be the only way you can go—and that's OK. Soups and liquid foods are a helpful ally when you are further along, and smaller meals eaten more frequently may relieve GI discomfort as your belly expands.

One of the kindest things you can do for yourself is become a master of anticipation. In an ideal world, having bland-but-settling bites stocked in your pantry, and gently nourishing soups prepared in your freezer, can be a huge boon, getting you through moments you just can't stomach cooking. And when your appetite revs back up—get ready! It can surprise you with its ferocity. Perhaps my biggest advice is to prep a snack or a full meal before you are ravenous; once that state hits, your mind can start to swim, and it is far harder to stay committed to a healthy choice—your brain will demand you fill up with whatever is on hand! Is there anyone else who you can ask to be the provider? Anticipating and feeding your hunger is one of the greatest acts of service to a mother-to-be; it's a great role to give to a partner who may be wondering what their part is in all this. Having a loved one anticipate your hunger and get cracking on a dish will become especially helpful as your pregnancy proceeds, when your ability to wait for mealtime might lessen dramatically.

2

Buffer the Worry

As you flip through the recipe section that follows, you may notice a bias toward cooked foods with lots of liquid involved. One of the reasons I'm so big on warm soups, broths, and stews, as well as cooked vegetables, is that these foods are easy for the body to digest. In Chinese medicine, the Stomach/Spleen is the epicenter of our digestive fire—it's like a cooking pot on a stove, heating and transforming ingredients you eat into energy and all the building blocks of life for baby and you. Throwing cold or icy food in this inner pot slows everything down, which can

Feeding Your Thyroid

One of the most under-supported parts of pregnant women's bodies is the thyroid gland, the master controller of metabolism in our bodies. Few know that we need to consciously feed it the raw materials it needs to make thyroid hormones, which means many people are going through pregnancy woefully depleted. You want to catch low thyroid function early and turn it around, for it not only compromises the baby's brain development, it can predispose you to postpartum struggles with weight, depression, future fertility, and more. One smart move is to make sure your diet contains adequate sources of iodine, the mineral that most helps this gland pump out these precious hormone messengers. I like to cook and eat with iodized sea salt, as well as seaweed and spirulina a few times during the week. Foods with high selenium content such as brazil nuts, cottage cheese, turkey, sunflower seeds, and sardines help the iodine get used by the thyroid, as does a healthy gut environment. Of course, a quality prenatal supplement will likely include both these minerals, but try to ensure your diet has enough of them too. Our wise ones suggest including comprehensive thyroid testing in your first trimester bloodwork panel, including testing for thyroid antibodies. Getting a jump on any thyroid dysfunction not only helps your baby, it can save you a lot of unnecessary suffering in the postpartum months.

cause digestive upset (gas, bloating, constipation) and stagnation in blood flow (making it harder for your organs to do their jobs), and then ripple upward to your state of mind as well. Wind in the body drives anxious, restless thoughts and contributes to over-worrying. So when you eat to keep heat in the Stomach and soothe and comfort the Spleen—and soupy foods are perfect for that as they're already cooked!—you can feel more grounded, calm, and warmed. During pregnancy, keeping this digestive fire well-tended helps keep your uterus (affectionately known as "the Baby Room" by my aunties) cozy and warm as well. As things start to get a little crowded in there, the bigger baby gets, your digestive system appreciates you helping it out with easy foods even more; your Liver and Spleen work hard to alchemize your food, but there's more pressure on them than before. Feel into how your meals are digesting and don't hesitate to lean on soft, warm, soupy, and liquid foods, like the soups and stews that follow, as well as my tried and tested Millet Ginger Congee (page 182).

Coffee Swaps

Sacrificing coffee can be hard for many. But don't despair! Delicious substitutes exist. At MotherBees, we like Rasa's herbal coffee alternatives, Four Sigmatic's mushroom blends, Vahdam Superfoods' turmeric latte mixes, and Teeccino, a tasty barley and chicory coffee alternative. Teeccino is great because it is a prebiotic as well as a coffee substitute. We also often drink hot chicken or fish broth in the morning to get the day going right!

Interestingly, the Spleen corresponds to the Earth element in the traditional Chinese view; it is the center of the five elements. Befitting its sun-like status, it likes foods with yellow and orange colors (which are often high in beta-carotene, a precursor to vitamin A), and an earthy, sweet taste—how perfect for this golden time of life! Some practitioners call the Spleen our inner child—it likes to feel safe and nurtured, not aggravated and edgy. If you have ever felt satiated and peaceful eating creamy mashed sweet potato lavished with grass-fed butter, or a steaming bowl of pho with noodles, or conversely thrown hangry tantrums when deprived of food for too long, now you know why. (Try the Coconut Kabocha & Red Lentil Soup, page 179). What the Spleen does not like are the foods you might turn to when feeling stressed and unsettled, like fried foods and fast food—these cause digestion to stagnate, and have unwanted inflammatory effects. The Spleen also finds big, protein-heavy meals at night a real burden to work with—so eat dinner a few hours before heading to bed, even if you need a small snack or some warm milk with ghee before eyes-closed time.

> A mother should not over-worry or think she's not doing a good job. For some people, when they are nauseous, they just cannot take the food. Eat when you can. Eat properly when there is no nausea.
>
> —DR. PADMA RAJU

Now, none of this means that cold foods or drinks are completely taboo when you're pregnant! In fact, during pregnancy and in the second trimester's growth spurts especially, you might want a counter-balance to the heat that naturally builds up inside from all the developmental activity. (Excess heat can be experienced as thirst, insomnia, night sweats, heartburn, constipation, and more.) Just how cold on the spectrum you can tolerate will depend on your constitution; everyone is different. Before you reach for very chilled foods and frosty drinks, see if cooling foods like cucumbers, jicama, celery, and watermelon can help temper the heat. Keep in mind that as a general rule, you want to keep your Stomach/Spleen happy by avoiding prolonged iciness in your belly.

3

Surround Yourself with Sweetness

I don't mean sugar in this instance! But rather, always remember to allow your food to make you happy. In my kitchen, that comes from enjoying the colors, textures, and aromas of my ingredients, and making the ambiance of my prep area uplifting and light-filled. (I even love to cut my vegetables in orderly sizes and shapes, then combine the colored cubes in painterly ways—even the peels in the sink look like strokes of color on a canvas to me!) Any time we awaken our senses, I think we feel more in touch with our life force—that blazing Shakti power of creation that rises up from the depths in this time. Colorful, flavorful food can be a balm for a tired spirit, if you take the time to notice. Sometimes we get so focused on meeting basic nutritional needs, we forget about pleasure. And even if the food you're eating is ultra-simple (perhaps even bland, if that's all you feel you want), the eating itself can become sweeter to the senses. Make a ritual of it. Even if you're alone, lay out a place mat and use your nicest bowl. Sink into your chair and let your shoulders relax with a long exhale. Notice the relief or even excitement that might flood through you knowing that food is ready. Put your fork down between bites and let your body be in peace. Eat until you are satiated—but not overly more than that, so your digestion can do its job. A short stroll after the meal helps the digestive chi descend and do its work, rather than ascend upwards, potentially causing heartburn and discomfort.

Perhaps my favorite way of all to surround with sweetness is to cook with others at my side. My family and I always notice how much better the food tastes when we have prepared it together, with one intention. After all, our cells vibrate with energetic frequency; having some "good vibes" in the kitchen seems to make even simple dishes more delicious and more digestible.

4

Claim Your Crown

Just like the commitment that you make to dig deep in order to give birth, there's a point where you decide, I'm going to do this. I'm going to make eating well a priority. And it comes when you stand in your power and decide: I deserve the best!, for no other reason than that you are becoming a Mother or Mother Again. Your deserving power is on high. In the kitchen, this looks a few ways. It starts by making some bold gestures to take control of your queendom and banishing the foods that might derail you from your pledge. Early on in pregnancy, I suggest clearing out any junk foods or drinks, or highly refined and nutrient-poor processed snack foods that might call to you when you're feeling tired or unprepared. Be bold— take your sword to them! Take just a short prep session where you look at packages, take inventory, and notice if these familiar foods are stripped of good nutrition or filled with too many sugars. They're the things you might default toward in wobbly, queasy moments, so it's helpful if they've gone away. Replace them with better alternatives. This sounds like a chore, but it can also be creative and fun! A lot of attention will soon go toward designing a nook or nursery for baby later in pregnancy, but why not start by curating your pantry or fridge, organizing its shelves and spaces with similar commitment and care?

The simple ingredients you'll see in the recipe pages that follow can cluster on them, bringing your healthy intentions to life. What's so beautiful is that as you bring in new, better provisions that match what you need in this time, your pantry starts to come alive with the essence of the new, evolving you! I also love to encourage mothers-to-be to notice the resistance that comes up around buying a few specialty ingredients that will serve in this time. It can feel hard to spend a few extra dollars on things specially for you. But funneling some of the grocery budget for your needs is warranted now; a helpful tip can be canceling one or two little-used media subscriptions and redirecting those small amounts to your food budget. It sets a new groove in place, no matter how small the amount. Some mothers like to start a pregnancy and postpartum savings account in their first weeks, squirreling extra funds into it—to the extent they can—so that they have a dedicated amount on hand for food and care that they don't feel shy about spending.

Claiming your crown also means practicing the art of asking for help and receiving. There is just no way around it. Preparing healthy meals takes effort and time—even when they're as ultra-simple as the ones that follow. It really is all hands on deck to keep the pregnant person well-resourced. And while you may not have extended family cooking for you, even if someone else in your home simply heats up the food you have previously cooked and refrigerated or frozen, or warms up a cup of broth from the fridge and hands it to you with a smile, you can gratefully receive. Small gestures like that go a long way toward avoiding depletion. Feeling taken care of ripples through you, nourishing and fortifying the body, mind, and spirit.

Invest in Yourself

We've been so conditioned that the pregnant woman is a do-it-all superwoman that it can be hard to notice the small ways you might get in the way of putting your good nourishment first. So ask yourself, do you feel worthy of spending the time, energy (or even the money) on your specific nourishment needs—even if they're a little different from other family members' needs? Do you feel deserving of help from others with shopping, cooking, or heck, cleaning the dishes? Do you pause and put your credit card back rather than splurge on that special, healing food item for yourself—the grass-fed ghee or manuka honey or bag of organic pumpkin seeds—even while your partner enjoys craft beer or cold brew coffee without a second thought? If you answer yes to any of these, it can be worth asking yourself why the resistance is coming up, and how would it feel to do differently? When you sit with these questions, you are committing to what I have come to learn is the deep inner work of mothering—putting a lid on the sabotaging voice saying you haven't done enough yet and grabbing even the smallest of moments to care deeply for yourself. You are, in a sense, encircling yourself with care, even when nobody else is around. Once you are in the thick of mothering, this skill of not abandoning yourself or your hunger becomes priceless. And there's no better time to get good at it than now.

No matter how much worthy nutritional advice you follow, always keep one truth in mind: No one knows your body better than you. In pregnancy, your instincts can get sharpened, and they can guide you now. You might notice a strong aversion to something your mind says you should eat. Likewise, a deep desire for something you didn't expect you'd ever want. These aversions and call-ings can be helpful signposts, and I believe in following them with a few caveats. (Interestingly, a yearning for sour foods early in pregnancy is seen by tradition-alists as the baby's Liver channel taking form—the Liver thrives with a touch of sour taste, and it is starting to kick into gear. So pay heed and crack open the sau-erkraut or slice into that grapefruit!)

The most obvious way to hone an intuitive approach to eating during preg-nancy is to eat when you are hungry; don't wait for an official mealtime hour. The next step is to notice how a meal makes you feel about an hour or two after eat-ing. I always want my meal to make me feel like I have got a light, warm blanket around my middle. Personally, when I eat raw food and chilled vegetables, or a cold banana or cheese right out of the fridge, my belly feels chilly. Soon, I notice bubbles of stress begin to move upward, as my mind starts to worry about an impend-ing tummy ache—belly and brain are that connected! My "warm belly/cold belly" is my own private and very simplified way of tuning into the Chinese tradition about warming and cooling foods (which to be frank, gets quite complex!). Cooling foods, like bananas and watermelon, and shrimp and crab, are considered to slow down circulation of Blood and chi, and they tend to be limited in pregnancy. Overly

Cravings, Decoded

Our wise ones, including my Auntie Ou, shared a beautiful sentiment. Starting in the second trimester, the baby whispers certain foods it needs to the mother in the form of cravings, to get her to consume certain nutrients it needs. If she completely denies them, it can cause more aggravation inside her body (and even cause the baby to want more of these foods later in life). I love this sentiment, in part because I love to tune in to the fact that babies don't lie, they communicate their express needs from the earliest moments, even in utero. Yet let's remember the old ways were not factoring in deep dish pizza or high fructose sweetened treats. By all means listen in to strong messages for certain foods, then layer in at least a moment of thoughtful pause, most especially if you're getting guided down the processed food or sweet treat aisle. Is this craving a real signpost, or a sign of something else? A deep yearning for sugar is often a cry for protein, so try that and a glass of water or herbal tea first.

heating foods like spicy and fried foods are said to cause internal fire that aggravates the fetus. A very basic way to explore this is in the morning. Start the day with some room temperature water, maybe with a slice of lemon. Then notice, are you feeling quite warm? Have some fruit for breakfast. Or are you feeling a little chilled? Then consume warming ginger tea, a bowl of congee (page 182) or even some fatty fish and avocado. Notice how you feel an hour after you eat. Do you feel good, settled, and at ease? Or not?

While an experienced practitioner of Chinese medicine might help you dial in pregnancy foods along these lines (tweaked according to your constitution and your phase of pregnancy), simply noticing how you feel after eating can tune you in to a finer level of feeling around food. Doing this is mothering in action—after all, once baby is here, we will watch her responses to each bite with an eagle eye, eager to make adjustments to keep her soothed and happy. Why not bring the same devoted care to ourselves?

Quick Kitchen Audit

Though there's a lot on your plate already when you are pregnant, it's a great time to clean up some basics to support you and your baby. If you don't filter your tap water, look into whatever level of filtration you can afford right now. (As mentioned in *The First Forty Days*, a good water filter can be an early "shower" gift for your family.) Look at how many plastic items you use or eat out of. Consider packing away all plastic cups and storage containers and replace them with glass jars. And audit your coated, nonstick pans; if you have any, are they scratched in any way? Scratched nonstick surfaces can easily leach very toxic chemicals into your food, which make their way to your baby in utero and into your breast milk. The safest bet is to switch over to ceramic or stainless-steel pans—and to use loads of butter or coconut oil on them to compensate for the lack of nonstick chemicals!

A MINIMALIST PREGNANCY PANTRY

There's nothing more reassuring than knowing you have the basics to put together a healthy meal, whether you are following a recipe or taking the most simple approach (like roast the squash, add butter and salt, then eat—see Roasted Sliced Kabocha Squash, page 195). Unlike some cooks, I appreciate a streamlined pantry and fridge because I get overwhelmed by too many bottles crammed on shelves or too much produce jammed into fridge drawers! Here are just a few of the foods to have on hand that I know will support you. As you flip through the recipes, keep these in mind as staples to shop for.

PLANT-RICH

Cabbages: red, green, napa

Cruciferous: arugula, bok choy, broccoli, broccolini, broccoli rabe, Brussels sprouts, cauliflower, collard greens, kale, kohlrabi, mustard greens, watercress

Greens: asparagus, beet green, celery, dandelion, endive, lettuce, spinach, Swiss chard

Mushrooms: beech, button, cremini, enoki, lion's mane, maitake, shiitake

Roots: beet, burdock, carrot, celeriac, daikon, fennel, garlic, ginger, onion, radish, sweet potato, turnip, white potato

FRUITS

Apple, apricot, avocado, banana (plantain), blackberry, blueberry, cranberry, cucumber, dragon fruit, figs (dry or fresh), gooseberry, grape, grapefruit, jujube (dry or fresh), lemon, mandarin, Medjool date, mulberry, papaya, pear (green, red, Asian), persimmon, prune, raisin, raspberry, watermelon, young coconut

NUTS & SEEDS

Nuts: almond, Brazil, cashew, macadamia, peanut, pistachio, walnut

Seeds: buckwheat, chia, flax, hemp, pine nuts, pomegranate, poppy, pumpkin, sesame, sunflower

PROTEINS

Bones: beef knuckle, beef marrow, chicken back, chicken feet, fish bone, oxtail

Land: beef, buffalo, chicken, egg, ground lamb, pork (whenever possible, fully grass-fed/pasture-raised and/or organic)

Ocean: anchovies, clam, herring, kipper, mackerel, mussel, oyster, salmon, scallop, shrimp, sole

OFFALS

Beef: heart, kidney, liver, oxtail, tongue, tripe

Chicken: gizzard, heart, liver

Lamb: heart, intestines, kidney, liver, tongue

Pork: blood, heart, intestines, kidney, liver, skin

Veal: brains, heart, kidney, liver, sweetbreads, tongue

CONDIMENTS
Black pepper, Bragg Liquid Aminos, coconut aminos, cumin powder, fish sauce, iodized sea salt, ketchup, nutritional yeast, tamari

FERMENTS
Kefir, kimchi, kombucha, miso, natto, pickled cucumbers, pickles, sauerkraut, sourdough, tempeh, yogurt

OILS
Avocado, coconut, grass-fed butter, extra-virgin olive, ghee, lard, sesame, tallow

DRY GOODS
Beans & Legumes: adzuki, black, black-eyed peas, cannellini, chickpeas, green peas, lentils (red, green, yellow), mung, navy, pinto

Grains: barley, millet, oats, quinoa

Powders: cacao, grass-fed collagen, Hawaiian spirulina, moringa, protein (organic whey, organic plant-based/green/hemp)

Rice: basmati, brown, black, jasmine, red, sweet (sticky) sushi

Seaweeds: hijiki, kombu, nori, wakame

DRIED HERBS FOR TEAS AND INFUSIONS
To ensure the utmost safety for you and your baby, obstetricians and midwives insist on knowing about any herbs, supplements, or over-the-counter medication that you may be taking. Though the herbs used in this book have centuries of safe use behind them, it is important to inform your doctor of any herbs that you would like to try.

Herbs: chamomile flowers, dandelion leaf, echinacea, lavender, lemon balm, milky oat, oat straw, peppermint leaf, red raspberry leaf, rose hip, rose petal, stinging nettle leaf

ACIDS
Apple cider vinegar, basmati vinegar, black vinegar, lemon juice, red vinegar, rice vinegar, ume plum vinegar, white vinegar, yuzu lemon juice

MILK PRODUCTS
Almond milk, cashew cheese, coconut cream, coconut milk, cottage cheese, cow milk, goat milk, hemp milk, macadamia milk, oat milk, rice milk

SWEETENERS
Allulose, brown cane sugar, honey, maple syrup, monk fruit, organic stevia, sunchoke

KITCHEN WISH LIST
Heavy-bottomed ceramic pots, food processor, glass storage containers, electric hot water kettle, high-speed blender, Instant Pot (many of the recipes can easily be adapted to pressure-cooking if you are familiar with this method), juicer, Mason jars (16 and 32 ounces/480 and 960 ml), measuring cup, measuring spoon, metal tongs, non-toxic nonstick skillet, parchment paper, rice cooker, slow cooker, strainer, steamer, tea strainer

ECO-FRIENDLY GROCERY SHOPPING WISH LIST
Basket, beeswax wrap (instead of foil or plastic wrap), reusable mesh produce bags, reusable shopping bags

Quick Home Remedies

Some of the most common discomforts of pregnancy can be aided or resolved with simple dietary and lifestyle measures. Try these simple tips.

Constipation: It's important to try to keep bowel movements regular. Initial hormone changes, and later your growing baby taking up space in utero, make constipation common. My acupuncturist, Dr. Hu, suggests eating plenty of cooked spinach with olive oil and salt; eating soaked raisins, prunes, and figs and drinking the soaking water; cooking with soft fruits (see Agni Stewed Apples & Prunes, page 213, and Beef Stew with Prunes, page 192); and lots of walking. My warm, soothing Millet Ginger Congee recipe, page 182, has a gently lubricating effect in the intestines, and I love cooked, mashed sweet potatoes (laden with coconut oil or butter!) for the same alleviating effect. Don't forget to feed your microbiome! Prebiotic foods and probiotic supplements can also help; many love adding a quality magnesium supplement too. Discuss this and further remedies with your care provider.

Nausea: As mentioned above, eat when you can. And if bland, carbohydrate-laden foods are all you can tolerate in those moments, give yourself some grace. (See if that settles your stomach enough to take in some protein and fat afterward.) Ginger is a time-tested nausea remedy—sip on the Asian Pear Ginger Tea (page 233). Another grandmother's kitchen trick is to scrape the peel of a lemon and smell its aroma. A few sips of the electrolyte drink called Recharge has helped many women through nausea—though I like making the homemade Morning Sickness Elixir on page 241. Sipping on low-sugar tonic water might also help in a pinch. And don't overlook Robin Lim's legendary Rujak (Indonesian Fruit Dip, page 225), which has helped countless women under her care. Keeping your magnesium levels up is also supportive. Wise one Karen Paul also recommends having a loved one grasp the nape of your neck and hold it for several minutes—this stimulates acupressure points that help alleviate the nausea. Homeopathic remedies for morning sickness include nux vomica 30c and pulsatilla 30c. As always, be sure to discuss with your care provider (ask about vitamin B6 supplementation) or find an experienced Chinese medicine practitioner for help if nausea becomes debilitating.

Heartburn: During pregnancy, the valve between stomach and esophagus relaxes, and this can sometimes let stomach acid leak back into the esophagus, causing heartburn. If this occurs, try eating smaller, more frequent meals, and avoid overly acidic foods. Fresh ripe papaya with a squeeze of lime juice or the Refreshing Papaya Smoothie on page 219 are good options. Papaya enzyme tablets can also help. Homeopathic remedies such as carbo vegetabilis (30c), or nux vomica (30c), may be used, also—a licensed homeopath or naturopath can really help relieve this issue.

Anemia: While anemia is common and not something to get scared about, it's something to treat so that fatigue, low immunity, and low spirits don't set in. Be sure to add iron-rich, blood building foods into your diet—try Coconut Apple Liver Pâté on page 210, Dragon Fruit Smoothie on page 223, Sesame Garlic Spinach on page 197, and Beet Cucumber Mint Juice on page 240, and sip on nettle infusion (like Stinging Nettle & Lemon Balm Tea, page 238) throughout the day. Make sure your prenatal vitamin contains sufficient iron in the form of non-constipating iron chelate, ideally, or talk to your provider about blood-building supplements.

Swelling: Late-pregnancy swelling has often been attributed to too much sodium in the diet; however, nutritional gurus like Dr. Tom Brewer describe how low protein levels are often the cause. Keep your hydration up and sip on the electrolyte-rich Morning Sickness Elixir, page 241, and Hydrating Berry Elixir, page 243. Cynthia Graham, a brilliant health counselor and dear friend of MotherBees, shares how with her pregnant clients, a short session of light exercise relieves swollen legs and feet with surprising ease.

Recipes

Whenever I cook for and with a mother-to-be, or with a new mom or her family, I don't get overly attached to what's in her fridge or on her cupboard shelves. I take a look and consider what I intuitively feel will nourish her best, and then assess: What do we have to work with today? In the ideal scenario, she's got a pantry fairly well supplied with provisions, which is the secret weapon to eating well. But even if something key is missing, or just ran out—because, well, life—I flow around that obstacle. It's all good. There is no shame in not having things perfectly lined up at all times! We'll just use something else.

Pregnancy and birth strip things down to their essence. Suddenly there you are, in active labor, naked or half naked, fully vulnerable and exposed as you and baby move through this passage—life in its pure essence, no frills or flourishes.

To that end, I believe the food you eat throughout pregnancy can be equally stripped down, most of the time. Make it simple, let good ingredients offer their benefits to you, and eat them in ways that make your digestion happy. It's enough. Sometimes we crack a cookbook, glance at the lists of ingredients we don't have on hand, and shut it, slightly ashamed. "Not today." I don't want that to happen in this instance. There should always be something that's a cinch to make, so that you never fall into moments of stress, doubt, or shame. To that end, you'll find some of these recipes to be almost monastically simple; a few ingredients put together simply, and using as few pots and pans as humanly possible. This is very much intentional! In this unpredictable time, ease and simplicity take on enormous new implications. Plus, your mind may be full of many considerations. If recipe steps remain uncomplicated, and you can simply be in your kitchen, breathing and being, I consider that a win.

My style of cooking is very intuitive. I'm not huge on ironclad rules or strict hard lines around food. So I've made these recipes open to wiggle room; they've got some space for your own hits of inspiration or they can mold to whatever you have on hand that day. Want to add an egg into your bowl of broth, to quickly whisk in more protein and fat . . . and then wilt some spinach in for easy cooked greens? Go for it! Want to make your congee plain, and top it with leftover chicken or fish from dinner last night? Your bowl and your belly will be happy you did! The very last thing I want you to feel is *There's nothing to eat*! So let yourself mix and match a little, adding ingredients and flavors if you feel confident (or curious) to do so. I'll offer a few suggestions for playing around as we go.

The recipes that follow are intended to be not only very easy to make, but ultra-inclusive. They give you a range of options that are plant-rich, meat-rich, and combinations of both. They offer alternatives to refined carbs and help nudge you away from overly blood-sugar–spiking meals. You will find lots of slow carb foods including a range of vegetables, roots, and tubers, and smaller portions of rice. (Know that you can always adjust the amount of rice, grains, etc. based on how your body is responding to pregnancy and what your trusted care provider recommends.) You may want to make double quantities of some recipes and freeze the extra for a future meal. A final note: I've offered an affirmation beneath each recipe. If it feels right to you, say it out loud a few times while you cook, or wash ingredients, or chop. It helps create that sweet moment of connection in the kitchen. Better yet, the words of wisdom might land and settle in you, until the moments—like the height of labor, or the depths of newborn-induced sleep deprivation—when you suddenly hear them again, reminding you of all that you are.

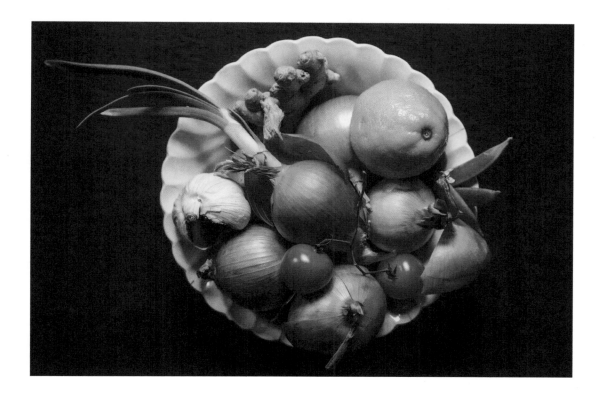

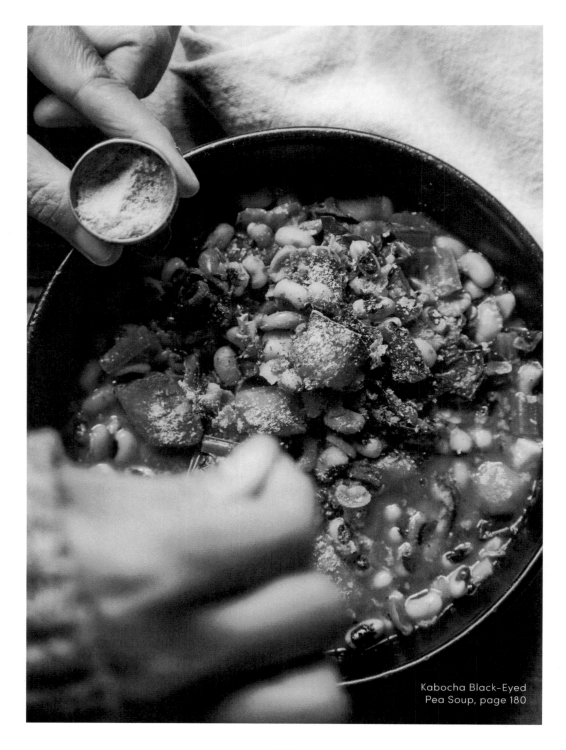

Kabocha Black-Eyed
Pea Soup, page 180

Note on Ingredient Sourcing

In terms of sourcing, I always aim to meet others where they are ideologically and financially. There has to be some wiggle room so meals fit your budget or your ability to source things easily. In a perfect world, I would wish for everyone on this planet to have access to vegetable and herb gardens fed by spring water and healthy, nutrient-rich soil, and to animal products that are raised to high standards of welfare and from regenerative farms (which help improve the environment and support rural communities). I do think pregnancy, a period of great change, is a great time to go that extra mile toward supporting farmers' markets and seeking fully grass-fed meats when you can. (You might be surprised that shopping this way can be more affordable than you think.) But when that's not in the cards, just make the next best choice you can. Likewise, be curious about the few unusual traditional ingredients included here and there—if you can source them, terrific, but if not, try the suggested substitutions. And please feel free to make tweaks that fit the way you eat—I've made a few suggestions, such as some interesting varieties of gluten-free noodles and some options for non-dairy milks. In the few places that cane sugar is used, you're welcome to try another sweetener, such as those listed in the Pantry section on pages 168–169. There are more choices now than ever before, so use your creativity to tailor my recipes as a foundation for what makes you feel your best!

It's often said that the more diverse a mom's palette during pregnancy, the more open her baby's palette will be for all kinds of foods—and having raised three adventurous eaters, I believe it. When picking fruits and veggies, go for the ones that are in season where you live—you'll get the most robust flavors, sweetness, and nutrition from the produce that hasn't been picked early and transported across continents. Finally, remember to always read your ingredient labels—the fewer and more familiar the ingredients, the better. (And take a brief pause to feel whether a particular food product is full of the nutrition your body needs, or empty of it—you might be surprised by what your intuition says!)

Don't hesitate to get support and advice from your trusted pregnancy care provider(s) on your diet too—if you're lucky, your practitioner may have a lot of good guidance to offer.

SOUPS, BROTHS & STEWS

Coconut Kabocha & Red Lentil Soup

This is a slightly revised version of my go-to postpartum soup—it is such a beautiful, simple, and healthy recipe, so I like to serve it to my pregnant mamas too. Kabocha squash is a personal favorite to use in my soups and stews. As it cooks, it breaks down into soft chunks that add a pleasing thick quality, as well as an array of vitamins, minerals, and fiber. I especially love it with the skin on, as it gives extra texture to the bite. Beautifully orange in color and slightly sweet in taste, this squash also pleases the Spleen, which helps support blood circulation to nourish the womb.

4 tablespoons (60 ml) avocado oil

1¼ teaspoons sea salt

½ (65 g) white onion, peeled, roughly chopped

1 tablespoon peeled and grated ginger

¼ teaspoon ground cumin

¼ teaspoon ground cinnamon

4 cups (635 g) kabocha squash, skin on, de-seeded, cut into ½-inch (12 mm) cubes (see Note)

2 quarts (2 L) cold water

1 cup (190 g) red lentils, rinsed

3 tablespoons coconut cream

4 tablespoons (44 g) nutritional yeast

black pepper to taste

In a large pot over medium heat, heat oil and ¼ teaspoon salt. Add onion and cook, stirring occasionally, for roughly 3 minutes, until lightly brown.

Add ginger, cumin, cinnamon, kabocha squash, and cold water. Bring to a boil, then turn down heat to medium-low, partially cover, and cook for 45 minutes.

Add red lentils, cook for 10 minutes, then stir in coconut cream and cook for another 10 minutes. Turn off the heat. Use a hand blender to give it a quick whirl or mash the kabocha squash with a fork until the soup is chunky.

Add nutritional yeast, 1 teaspoon salt, and pepper to taste.

Note: Cutting kabocha squash is a pain, so consider this tip. Puncture the squash several times with a sharp knife and microwave for 4 to 5 minutes, then let cool slightly before cutting.

SOUPS, BROTHS & STEWS

Serves 6

I am deeply grateful for what I have today.

Kabocha Black-Eyed Pea Soup

In the American South, black-eyed peas are a staple for many dishes, especially around New Year's Day, as they are a symbol of good luck. Similarly, this ingredient is a Southern mother's favorite for before and after birth. Black-eyed peas normally appear light yellow in color with a black spot (hence the name), and one cup provides 52 percent of the recommended daily intake of folate. This aids greatly in producing enough red blood cells to avoid developing anemia during pregnancy.

1 cup (170 g) dry black-eyed peas

1 strip dry kombu seaweed

3 tablespoons apple cider vinegar

13 cups (3.2 L) cold water

4 garlic cloves

2 cups (320 g) kabocha squash, skin on, cut into 1-inch (2.5 cm) cubes

4 cups (140 g) roughly chopped Swiss chard

2 tablespoons nutritional yeast

sea salt and black pepper to taste

Soak black-eyed peas, kombu seaweed, and 1 tablespoon of apple cider vinegar in 5 cups (1.2 L) cold water overnight. Strain and rinse well under fresh running water.

In a large pot, add 8 cups (2 L) cold water and strained black-eyed peas, kombu seaweed, and garlic cloves. Bring to a boil, then turn down heat to medium-low, partially cover, and cook for 45 minutes.

After the peas are soft, add kabocha squash and cook for another 40 minutes.

Add chard and let cook for another 20 minutes. Turn off the heat and stir in the remaining 2 tablespoons apple cider vinegar and nutritional yeast. Season with salt and pepper to taste, and serve.

Serves 6

My voice matters.

Mung Bean Porridge

Tiny green mung beans have an ancient legacy. They've been noted in Asian cuisine as early as 1500 BCE! High in folate, protein, calcium, and iron, in Chinese medicine it is said that they aid with blood production, helping counter anemia. According to TCM, mung beans are "cold" (yin), as they help dispel internal heat and clear toxins from both mom and baby. This is a simple, light porridge that can be eaten on its own or amped up in flavor with any of the toppings from Millet Ginger Congee (page 182).

1 teaspoon sesame oil

3 tablespoons (38 g) sprouted mung beans

2 tablespoons (23 g) white jasmine rice

2 tablespoons (23 g) sweet (sticky) sushi rice

3½ cups (840 ml) cold water, Golden Chicken Ginger Broth (page 185), or other broth of choice

1 teaspoon ghee

sea salt to taste

OPTIONAL
sauerkraut

sesame seeds

In a medium pot over medium heat, add oil, mung beans, and rice. Cook, stirring often, for about 2 minutes until rice becomes translucent.

Add 3 cups (720 ml) cold water or broth and simmer over medium heat for 20 minutes, partially covered to ensure it does not boil over, stirring often. Reduce the heat to low, add an additional ½ cup (120 ml) cold water and cook for another 30 minutes. Season with ghee and salt to taste, top with sauerkraut and sesame seeds (if using), and serve warm.

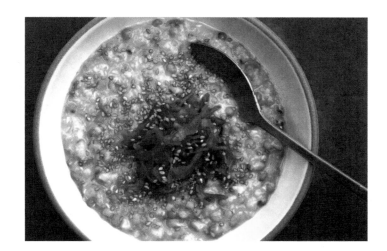

Serves 2

My life is precious. My baby's life is precious.

SOUPS, BROTHS & STEWS

Millet Ginger Congee

Congee, or rice porridge, is traditionally eaten in Asia as a breakfast dish. It is often made from leftover rice cooked with more water or broth the next day, but for this recipe, we are starting with uncooked rice and millet. A bowl of congee feels soft, simple, and soothing—I consider it edible comfort for the belly and soul, which is especially helpful if you are feeling nauseated. This dish's neutral flavor and light hint of ginger make it a winner when your appetite is curbed and your belly feels rather blah. Its lubricating moistness also helps keep elimination regular. If you want just plain congee, omit the ginger. Customize this base recipe with toppings per your taste.

2 tablespoons (23 g) white jasmine rice

2 tablespoons (23 g) sweet (sticky) sushi rice

3 tablespoons (30 g) millet grain

1 (2-inch/5 cm) knob fresh ginger, skin on, halved

3 cups (720 ml) cold water, Golden Chicken Ginger Broth (page 185), or other broth of choice

In a medium pot over medium-high heat, combine jasmine and sushi rice, millet, ginger, and 3 cups (720 ml) cold water or broth. Bring to a boil, about 20 minutes, then reduce the heat to low for 1 hour, stirring occasionally. Set a timer.

To serve, enjoy plain or with suggested toppings below.

Optional flavorings: Bragg Liquid Aminos, coconut aminos, fish sauce, sea salt

Optional toppings: Extra shredded chicken from Chicken Ginger Rice Soup (page 186), Roasted Sliced Kabocha Squash (page 195), Garlic Broccoli Rabe (page 196), Sesame Garlic Spinach (page 197), Powerhouse Mushroom Medley (page 199), Savory Zucchini Dill Fritters (page 200), Garlic-Butter Steak Bites (page 206), fried egg, kimchee, pickles, sauerkraut

Serves 2

I celebrate small victories daily.

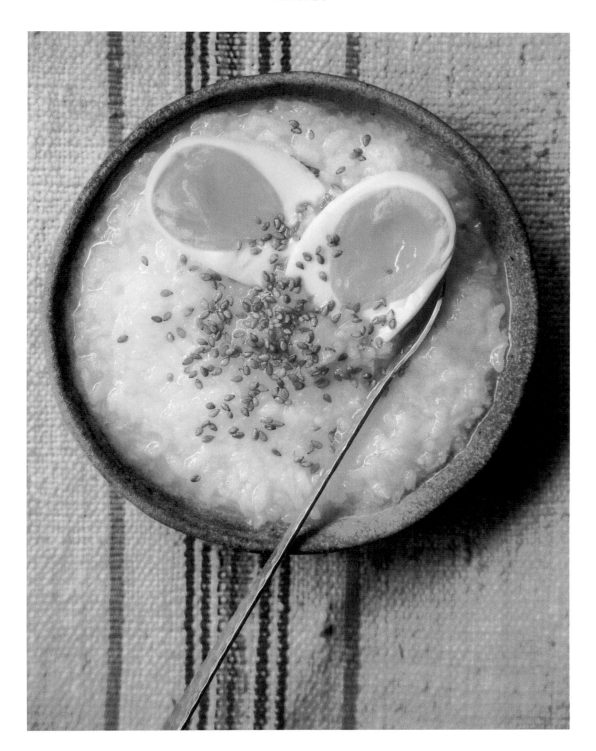

Salmon Head Broth

In Chinese medicine, salmon is seen to strengthen the Spleen, enhance chi (your vital life force), and remove dampness that can slow digestion and make you feel lethargic (like you're dragging). The bones, heads, cartilage, and fat from fish like salmon are super supportive during pregnancy thanks to their high levels of calcium, iron, zinc, omega-3 fatty acids, and gelatin (with all that fabulous glycine). Not only do they build up the mother's health (and give her glowing skin), they supercharge the baby's developing brain—motivating many a Chinese auntie or grandmother to reserve precious fish heads for the mother-to-be! Ask the fishmonger at your local store for them. These overlooked parts of fish, so often tossed out today, really prove their worth in this simple, warming broth. Try it in the morning when you crave a comforting hot drink that gives you a lift.

1 tablespoon avocado oil

1 (120 g) white onion, halved

1 (1-inch/2.5 cm) knob fresh ginger, skin on, sliced

2 garlic cloves, crushed with the flat side of a knife

1 large (375 g) tomato, quartered

3 fresh salmon heads (2 pounds/1 kg total), gills removed, rinsed

¼ teaspoon fennel seeds

2 quarts (2 L) cold water

3 green onions, whole

1 teaspoon sea salt to taste

Heat oil in a large pot over medium heat. Lightly brown the white onion, ginger, and garlic for 10 minutes, stirring occasionally.

Add tomato and let cook for an additional 2 minutes.

Add fish heads, fennel seeds, and cold water. Simmer over medium heat for 2 hours, skimming off the top layer of scum with a spoon.

During the last 10 minutes, add green onions and salt. Strain broth and eat fish head meat (optional).

Freezing tip: Fill two 16-ounce (480 ml) glass Mason jars or one 32-ounce (960 ml) glass Mason jar, leaving about 1 inch (2.5 cm) of room at the top, and place in the freezer, without lids. Once frozen, place the lids on. This will prevent the glass from cracking. Freeze for up to 2 months.

Serves 4

I am nourishing my body and my baby.

Golden Chicken Ginger Broth

This is an easy recipe that can be used as a cooking stock or sipped as a broth. It's such a breeze to make; consider cooking it every Sunday to have on hand throughout the week. The choice is yours: Add it to your veggie sautés; create instant noodle soups with rice noodles, egg, and spinach; or just season a mug of it with lemon juice, fish sauce, or soy sauce and sip. I encourage you to add the chicken feet here, because the boost of collagen they provide will help your skin's elasticity—all around your growing belly, and later, your perineum, which must stretch during labor and delivery. (Side note: Massaging the perineum with organic coconut oil during the last few weeks of pregnancy helps further!) Drinking this golden broth daily can really help if you are told you are low in amniotic fluid during your third trimester. Ask the butcher at your local grocery about ordering chicken backs and feet—many good stores can do that for you.

3 pounds (1.4 kg) chicken backs

1 pound (455 g) chicken feet

7 quarts (6.6 L) cold water

3 (2-inch/5 cm) knobs fresh ginger, skin on, sliced

1 teaspoon sea salt to taste

To prepare the chicken backs and feet for the broth, first clean them in the traditional way: In a large pot, add the backs and feet. Fill with 3 quarts (2.8 L) cold water and bring to a quick boil over medium heat for 30 minutes. Strain and discard the water, then rinse the chicken bones several times with fresh water until the water runs clear.

Return the chicken to the pot with another 4 quarts (3.8 L) cold water, add the ginger, and heat over medium-high. Bring to a boil, around 30 minutes, reduce the heat to medium-low, and cook for 3 hours, partially covered, skimming off the top layer of scum with a spoon.

It's finished! Strain the broth and add salt to taste. Once cooled, store in glass containers in the fridge and use throughout the week.

Note: If you feel like chopping veggies, you can add onion, carrots, celery, or herbs of your choice to bring another layer of flavor in. If you don't feel like it, the essentials above will do the job.

Serves 6 to 8

I embrace support and continue to set safe boundaries for myself.

Chicken Ginger Rice Soup

My deep fascination with perinatal biology began way back in high school. Among many incredible facts, I remember learning that at ten weeks, the fetus begins to produce urine which is secreted into the amniotic sac—wow! As an adult, I researched more to learn that during the second and third trimesters, as the amniotic fluid expands and baby's kidneys begin to function, fetal urine becomes the largest source of amniotic fluid. Lung secretions and gastrointestinal excretions from the umbilical cord and placenta also contribute to the composition. By late pregnancy, the fluid is clear or straw-colored, comprising 98 percent water plus electrolytes, peptides, carbohydrates, lipids, and hormones. In order for the baby to urinate often, the pregnant mom needs to consume lots of liquids, hence this Chicken Ginger Rice Soup. Drink this often late in pregnancy, several cups a week, to maintain a healthy amount of fluid.

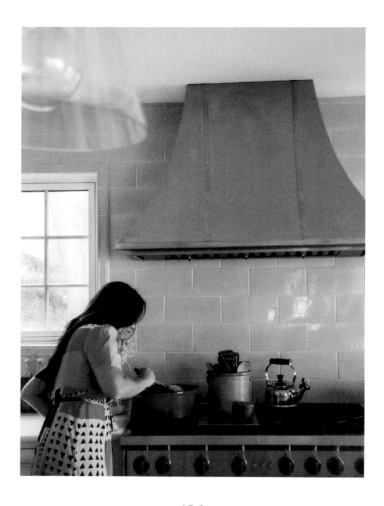

1 whole chicken
(4.3 pounds/1.95 kg),
rinsed, giblets bag removed

6 quarts (5.7 L) plus 1 cup
(240 ml) cold water

¼ cup (50 g) jasmine rice

¼ cup (50 g) sweet (sticky)
sushi rice

2 (2-inch/5 cm) knobs fresh
ginger, skin on, sliced

2 teaspoons sea salt

OPTIONAL

½ teaspoon fish sauce per
serving

scallions, thinly sliced

To prepare the chicken, first clean it in the traditional way: In a large pot, add the whole chicken. Fill with 3 quarts (2.8 L) cold water and bring to a quick boil over medium heat for 30 minutes. Strain and discard the water, then rinse the chicken several times with fresh water until the water runs clear.

Return the chicken to the pot with another 3 quarts (2.8 L) cold water and heat over medium, partially covered. Bring to a soft boil and cook for about 30 minutes.

Meanwhile, in a small bowl, combine jasmine rice, sushi rice, and 1 cup (240 ml) cold water. Set aside to soak.

Using tongs, remove the chicken from the pot and place it on a large baking sheet. Use two forks to pull apart the soft, cooked chicken meat and set aside or store; save for Rich & Creamy Noodles with Vegetables (page 201) or to top your Millet Ginger Congee (page 182).

Add the carcass and bones back into the broth and cook over medium heat for 40 more minutes. Strain the bones and discard, then add the liquid broth back into the pot.

Strain and rinse the soaked rice.

Add rice and ginger slices to the broth. Cook over medium-low for another 40 minutes, stirring often—remember to set a timer. When the soup is finished, stir in the salt.

Serve with a dash of fish sauce and scallions (if using).

Serves 6 to 8

I am creating a bountiful home for my baby to grow in.

Nourishing Lotus Root Seaweed Soup

At MotherBees, when great quality pork bones are available and lotus root is in season, this simple soup is constantly stewing on my stovetop—I love how its combination of pork, seaweed, lotus root, ginger, and goji berries works to replenish the body's vital life force, known as chi. It is gently fortifying! May this recipe tempt you to start the rhythmic ritual of making soup weekly: You come home from the market, throw ingredients in a pot, and let it cook. Better yet, this soup invites you to linger at the table, dipping succulent flakes of meat into a tasty side sauce. Maybe it should be called "slow-down soup" for that reason. And if you're wondering, lotus root is the root of the gorgeous lotus flower, famed for eons as a symbol of personal illumination. You can find it in most Asian grocery stores—its vitamin C, mineral, and fiber content add to the great nourishment from the pork, seaweed, and broth. Traditionally, we serve rib bones and chunks of pork in each bowl, then pull meat off the bones as we go, dipping it in dunking sauce as we drink the soup. If you prefer, you can take out the rib bones, remove the meat, and place it back into the soup, discarding the bones before serving.

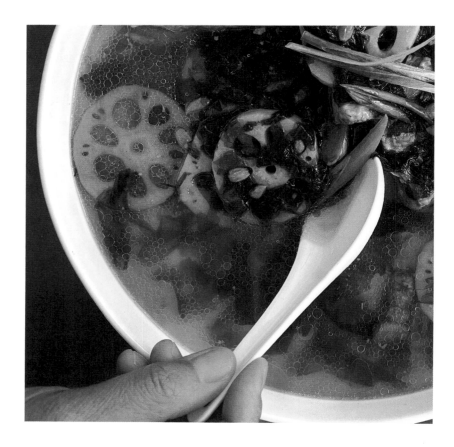

4 tablespoons (14 g) dry wakame seaweed

4 quarts (3.8 L) plus 1 cup (240 ml) cold water

1 pound (455 g) pork ribs, cut into individual ribs

1 pound (455 g) pork butt, cut into 2-inch (5 cm) cubes

1 small (13 g) lotus root, washed, peeled, and sliced ¼ inch (6 mm) thick

1 (2-inch/5 cm) knob fresh ginger, skin on, sliced

1 teaspoon goji berries

½ teaspoon sea salt

DIPPING SAUCE

2 tablespoons peeled and finely chopped white onion

3 tablespoons soy sauce (substitution: Bragg Liquid Aminos or gluten-free tamari)

2 tablespoons vinegar (options: black vinegar, apple cider vinegar, white vinegar)

1 tablespoon sesame oil

1 teaspoon cane sugar

Soak the wakame seaweed in 1 cup (240 ml) cold water for 20 minutes. Strain and rinse, then set aside.

To prepare the pork for the soup, first clean it in the traditional way: In a large pot, add the pork ribs and butt. Fill with 2 quarts (2 L) cold water and bring to a quick boil over medium-high heat for 15 minutes. Strain and discard the water, then rinse the meat several times with fresh water until the water runs clear.

Return the meat to the same large pot. Add the wakame, lotus root, ginger, and 2 quarts (2 L) cold water. Bring to a boil over medium-high heat for 15 minutes. Turn the heat down to a low simmer, partially cover, and cook for 1½ hours.

When 15 minutes remain, add the goji berries and continue simmering.

Meanwhile, prepare the dipping sauce by combining all sauce ingredients in a small bowl; set aside.

Now it's ready to eat. Turn off the heat and add salt to taste. Dip the meat into the dipping sauce.

Pro tip: Cooling and storing the soup in the fridge for a day before eating will concentrate the flavors.

SOUPS, BROTHS & STEWS

Serves 8

I can receive support mentally, physically, and spiritually.

189

Hearty White Bean Pork Stew

I love the hearty, filling, and warming qualities of this deeply nourishing stew. It's such a perfect mix of fortifying and health-giving foods in one bowl, and so easy to make too. This is one of my favorite dishes to make when visiting a mother-to-be's home. I place all the ingredients into a large pot without much fanfare as we have a heart-to-heart; and I can leave knowing the soup will cook on, making a delicious meal for her and her family. When I eat this soup, my cheeks get rosy and my body fills with energy as the protein and enriching fat from the pork delivers sustenance to my cells. See if you notice this happening for you.

1 pound (455 g) pork ribs, cut into individual ribs

1 pound (455 g) pork butt, cut into 2-inch (5 cm) cubes

3½ quarts (3.4 L) cold water

2 tablespoons avocado oil

½ (55 g) white onion, peeled, roughly chopped

1 medium leek, white part only, sliced into semicircles

2 small garlic cloves, roughly chopped

½ teaspoon ground cumin

1 (29-ounce/822 g) can cannellini beans, strained, rinsed

2 cups (70 g) Swiss chard or collard greens, roughly chopped

1 to 2 teaspoons sea salt

squeeze of lemon juice

To prepare the pork for the soup, first clean it in the traditional way: In a large pot, add the meat. Fill with 2 quarts (2 L) cold water and bring to a quick boil over medium-high heat for 15 minutes. Strain and discard the water, then rinse the meat several times with fresh water until the water runs clear. Set aside on a plate.

In the same large pot, heat oil over medium-high. Add the onion, leek, garlic, and cumin and cook, stirring occasionally, for roughly 10 minutes, until lightly brown.

Add the meat to the caramelized aromatics, pour in 1½ quarts (1.4 L) cold water, and bring to a boil for 15 minutes.

Add the beans and simmer over medium-low, partially covered, for an additional 1 hour.

In the last 10 minutes, stir in the greens and cook until soft but still a vibrant green color.

Season to taste with salt and serve with a squeeze of lemon.

Serves 8

I take one full breath at a time.

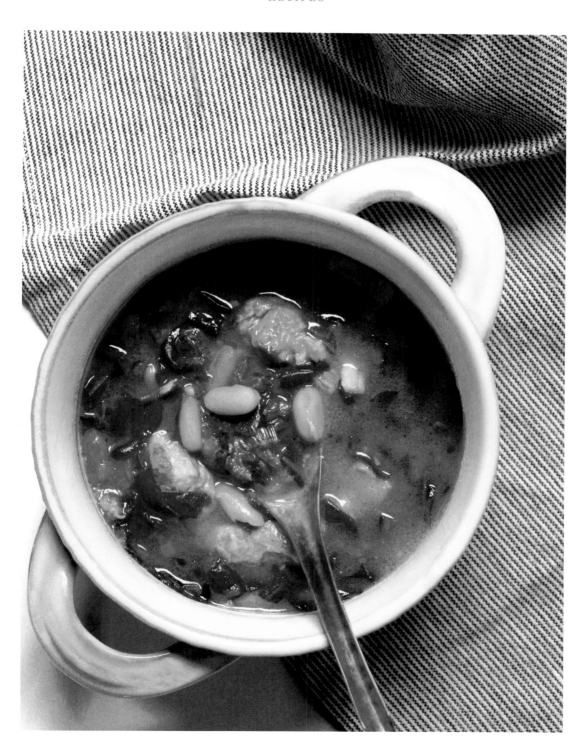

Beef Stew with Prunes

When I was pregnant back in my London days, I reveled in how well-versed local butchers were about their meat sources, including how they were raised, and how best to cook each cut. I miss this kind of personal shopping experience! If meat and prunes give you pause, know that this combination is common in traditional cooking across Asia and the Middle East. The fruit softens during cooking and releases its juices, infusing a rich flavor into the stew and thickening the liquid for extra texture. If you are able to source fully grass-fed beef from a producer that follows regenerative agriculture principles, that's even better! You're supporting the environment and local farming as you boost your family's health.

2 pounds (1 kg) boneless beef, preferably chuck stew meat, cut into 2-inch (5 cm) cubes

½ teaspoon sea salt, plus more to taste

½ teaspoon ground black pepper, plus more to taste

5 tablespoons (75 ml) avocado oil

1 (160 g) white onion, peeled, roughly chopped

2 tablespoons tomato paste

¼ teaspoon ground cinnamon

2 star anise pods

3 cups (720 ml) cold water or stock of choice

2 tablespoons soy sauce (substitution: Bragg Liquid Aminos or gluten-free tamari)

1 cup (250 g) prunes, pitted

1 (2-inch/5 cm) knob fresh ginger, skin on, sliced

Season beef cubes with salt and pepper and, if needed, separate into two batches for browning. In a large, heavy-bottom pot over medium-high heat, add 2 tablespoons avocado oil per batch and brown meat on all sides without stacking, about 4 minutes. When all the beef is browned, set aside on a large plate.

In the same pot over medium-high heat, add the remaining 1 tablespoon oil, the onion, and a little salt and lightly brown for 3 minutes.

Turn heat down to medium-low and add the tomato paste, cinnamon, star anise, cold water or stock, soy sauce, prunes, ginger and the browned meat. Bring back to a slow boil over medium heat, partially covered, then reduce to a low simmer. Cook for 2 hours, stirring occasionally. Set a timer. Season with salt and pepper to taste.

Serves 6 to 8

I am unique.

Star Anise Oxtail Stew

There may be days during your pregnancy when your body aches, your mood shifts, and the uncertainty about what's to come rattles your footing. If so, turn to this grounding, nutrient-dense recipe! I love using oxtail—it's quite old-school and it reminds me of the matriarchs in my family kitchens. This dish might take a few hours to cook, but the aroma that floats through the house might just give you a sense of ease and calmness, not to mention the pleasure of gnawing on the delicious, finger-licking bones.

3 pounds (1.4 kg) oxtail bones

4 quarts (3.8 L) cold water

1 (2-inch/5 cm) knob fresh ginger, skin on, sliced

1 pod star anise

2 bay leaves

4 garlic cloves

1 large tomato, quartered

1 large white potato, any variety, peeled, cubed

1 to 2 teaspoons sea salt

black pepper to taste

To prepare the oxtail bones for the soup, first clean them in the traditional way: In a large pot, add the oxtail bones. Fill with 2 quarts (2 L) cold water and bring to a quick boil over medium-high heat for 15 minutes. Strain and discard the water, then rinse the oxtail bones several times with fresh water until the water runs clear.

In the same large pot with the oxtail bones, add ginger, star anise, bay leaves, garlic, and 2 quarts (2 L) cold water. Partially cover the pot and bring to a quick boil over high heat for 25 minutes, then turn the heat down to medium-low. After 1 hour, add the tomato and potato and cook for another 3 hours. Add salt and pepper to taste.

Serves 6

I am feeding my baby nourishing foods and nourishing thoughts.

VEGETABLES

Roasted Sliced Kabocha Squash

During pregnancy, it is not at all uncommon for your digestion to get stuck and for constipation to set in. Including this fiber-rich squash in your diet, along with drinking enough fluids, can often get things moving down there pretty quickly. Kabocha is flavorful, filling, and chock-full of good nutrients such as beta carotene, vitamin C, iron, and calcium. It tastes a little like pumpkin, sweet potato, and chestnuts mixed together—sweet and savory—and it has a soft but thick texture. I personally love to eat the skin, so I always scrub it well before cooking! Having roasted squash slices ready to go in your fridge means that you can easily grab a couple slices to top your rice porridge. Add a fried egg and some leftovers from the night before to create a simple bowl.

1 medium (2.5 pounds/
1.2 kg) kabocha squash
(see Note, page 179)

⅓ cup (75 ml) avocado oil

½ teaspoon sea salt

black pepper to taste

4 whole garlic cloves,
unpeeled

Preheat the oven to 400°F (204°C).

Wash the kabocha, then use a large knife to cut it in half from top to bottom, avoiding the hard stems. Pull out the seeds and discard. Cut the halves, skin on, into 1-inch- (2.5 cm) thick slices.

In a large mixing bowl, combine all ingredients with your hands.

Cover a large baking sheet with parchment paper and transfer the mixed contents onto the sheet, laying each slice on its side, without stacking. Place in the oven and bake for 30 minutes. Set a timer.

The kabocha is ready when the edges are brown and the outer skin is bubbled a little. Enjoy warm!

VEGETABLES

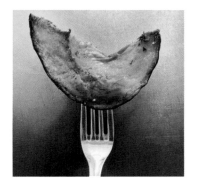

Serves 4

I am proud of my body.

Garlic Broccoli Rabe

One of my favorite vegetables, broccoli rabe (also known as rapini) has a nice bite and chew, and a slight yet pleasant bittersweetness. I find it much more tasty than straight broccoli. Since you want to eat several servings of vegetables every day—and please, not just cold-from-the-fridge salad leaves—this is a great way to load your bowl or plate with darker green vegetables full of fiber. Broccoli rabe is quite high in iron too. Try adding this to your bowl of Garlic-Butter Steak Bites (page 206) or your serving of Millet Ginger Congee (page 182). Eat it often enough while pregnant, and later on your baby might have quite a taste for it too.

2 quarts (2 L) cold water

1 teaspoon sea salt, plus more to taste

1 bunch (8 ounces/227 g) broccoli rabe, cut in half

1 tablespoon avocado oil

1 garlic clove, minced

1 tablespoon butter or ghee (substitution: vegan butter—I recommend Miyoko's Creamery)

black pepper to taste

In a medium pot over medium-high heat, bring 2 quarts (2 L) cold water and salt to a boil. Add broccoli rabe and cook for 5 minutes, or until stems are medium soft, then strain and run under fresh water.

In the same medium pot, heat avocado oil over medium. Add garlic and lightly brown for 1 minute.

Add butter and broccoli rabe and toss to coat for 1 minute. Season to taste with salt and pepper, stir, and enjoy.

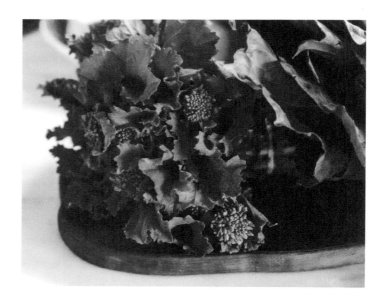

Serves 2

My baby and I are loved, nourished, and thriving in golden light.

Sesame Garlic Spinach

Eating spinach or other dark leafy greens is especially important during the first and second trimester. In Chinese medicine, spinach is considered a "reinforcement food," meaning it gives extra support to the organs and systems in your body that are working hard to make your baby. I add a splash of yuzu juice for its tangy fragrance, but if you don't have that, you can use ordinary lemon juice. Yuzu is a citrus fruit prized for its ability to alleviate inflammation, inhibit blood clotting, and boost the immune system. Personally, just smelling yuzu enhances my mood, and I think it may well do the same for you.

4 quarts (3.8 L) cold water

1 tablespoon sea salt

2 bunches (16 ounces/455 g) spinach, rinsed well (keep pink ends for extra sweetness)

2 tablespoons sesame oil

1 garlic clove, minced

2 tablespoons sesame seeds

1 tablespoon soy sauce (substitution: Bragg Liquid Aminos or gluten-free tamari)

1 tablespoon lemon juice

OPTIONAL
1 tablespoon yuzu juice (found in Japanese grocers or online)

In a large mixing bowl, make an ice bath with ice cubes and water and set aside. (If you want to skip this step, rinse spinach under cold running water after blanching.)

In a large pot over medium-high heat, bring cold water and salt to a boil. Add spinach and cook for 1½ minutes to blanch.

Strain spinach, then place in the ice bath for 1 minute (or rinse under cold running water), as this will maintain the vibrant green color.

Squeeze out excess water and form the spinach into a ball, then cut into quarters.

In the same large pot, heat the sesame oil, add the garlic and sesame seeds, and lightly brown over medium heat for 1 minute.

Turn off the heat and mix in the spinach, soy sauce, lemon juice, and yuzu juice (if using).

VEGETABLES

Serves 6

I am in charge of my life and my body.

Cauliflower Millet Mash

Cauliflower is a cruciferous vegetable, rich in folate and other minerals and antioxidants beneficial for fetal development. With 11 percent of your daily choline intake in one cup, cauliflower is one of the best plant-based sources of this super important nutrient. Choline, pronounced "ko-leen," is essential to developing a baby's spinal cord, and studies show significant cognitive benefits in the offspring of pregnant women who consume close to twice the recommended amount of choline (450 mg) daily during their last trimester. That's a lot of cauliflower! Millet is in the recipe as a naturally gluten-free grain, rich in dietary fiber, and also known as a prebiotic. It might take a little time to cook, but once it does, it becomes soft and easy to mash, which is fitting for this dish.

3 cups (720 ml) cold water

2 cups (215 g) roughly chopped cauliflower, or "riced" cauliflower

½ cup (100 g) millet, rinsed

½ teaspoon sea salt

¼ cup (15 g) nutritional yeast

1 tablespoon lemon juice

¼ cup (25 g) grated Parmesan cheese

In a medium pot over medium-high heat, bring cold water to a boil, then add cauliflower, millet, and salt. Reduce the heat to medium-low and cook for 30 minutes, stirring often so the millet doesn't stick to the bottom of the pot, until water is cooked down and the millet is soft.

When the millet and cauliflower are soft like mashed potato, take the pot off the heat. Using a fork, mix in nutritional yeast and lemon juice, then let it stand for 5 minutes. Fold in the grated Parmesan before serving.

Serves 4

I am present in my body. I honor my uterus, placenta, umbilical cord, and my baby.

Powerhouse Mushroom Medley

I recommend pairing this satisfying dish with scrambled eggs, scooped next to Savory Zucchini Dill Fritters (page 200), or with Sesame Garlic Spinach (page 197). Many people forget about using mushrooms regularly, but they are a powerhouse of nutrients including iron, vitamins B and D, and several key minerals that support your baby's development. I especially love shiitake mushrooms for their immunity-supporting effects. Most healthy grocery stores will carry a variety of mushrooms including the beech mushroom, which looks like a larger enoki and comes in white or brown varieties. If you have trouble sourcing all the mushrooms suggested here, feel free to substitute roughly chopped cremini mushrooms as needed. Another favorite mushroom of mine for brain power is the white, furry lion's mane mushroom found in farmer's markets or natural food markets. Try some sliced and cooked with butter in a hot pan!

3 tablespoons avocado oil, coconut oil, or ghee

2 cups (195 g) shiitake or 2 cups (120 g) cremini mushrooms, roughly chopped

2 cups (120 g) beech mushrooms, roughly chopped

2 garlic cloves, minced

sea salt and black pepper to taste

In a large nonstick pan, heat oil over medium-high. Wait until the pan is very hot, then add mushrooms and garlic. Brown mushrooms on both sides, trying not to stack them.

Add salt and pepper to taste.

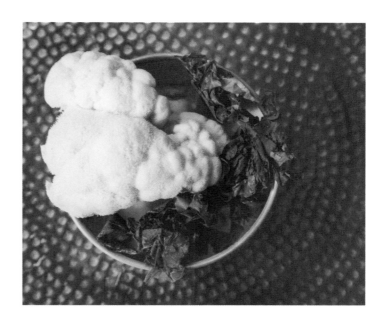

VEGETABLES

Serves 2 or 3

I am open to receiving all things good.

Savory Zucchini Dill Fritters

In the West, we prize certain vegetables for all the minerals and fiber they contain; in Chinese medicine, they're also prized for their cooling effects on the body. This can be helpful as you move into your second trimester, when the increase in blood circulation can create excess heat (which you might experience as excessive thirst, flushing, insomnia, night sweats, heartburn, and constipation). Zucchini, along with other cooling foods like mushrooms, asparagus, broccoli, and artichoke, can help counterbalance this effect. Though a simple steam with salt and butter will get you there quickly, try these fritters if you have just a little more time—they're very much a California twist on the old wisdom, and they also hit the spot if you're craving something fried! Any children in your household will also love to munch on them.

2 cups (230 g) grated zucchini

½ cup (55 g) peeled, finely chopped white onion

1 garlic clove, minced

2 tablespoons fresh dill, finely chopped

1 tablespoon nutritional yeast

large pinch sea salt and black pepper

1 tablespoon coconut flour

2 eggs, whisked

3 tablespoons avocado oil

Line a bowl with a clean kitchen towel. Place grated zucchini on the towel, then squeeze out all the extra liquid. Transfer zucchini to a large bowl.

Add onion, garlic, dill, nutritional yeast, salt, and pepper, then sift in coconut flour to avoid clumping.

Add whisked eggs and combine.

Heat a large nonstick pan over medium heat. When hot, coat the bottom of the pan with oil and heat for another minute.

Working in two batches, three fritters at a time, spoon ¼ cup (60 ml) of the mixture into the pan, flattening with a spatula. Cook for 3 to 4 minutes on each side until golden brown.

Serves 2 (yields 6)

I am making great food choices for myself and my baby.

Rich & Creamy Noodles with Vegetables

Although you don't want to lean on carb-heavy pastas and noodles when you're pregnant, sometimes they are exactly what you crave. This recipe is my healthy way to satiate the desire. I've added peanut butter to cream up the sauce, and you can add more veggies or the shredded chicken from Chicken Ginger Rice Soup (page 186).

NOODLE SAUCE

2 tablespoons organic peanut or almond butter

1½ tablespoons soy sauce (substitution: Bragg Liquid Aminos or gluten-free tamari)

1 tablespoon sesame oil

½ teaspoon cane sugar

⸺

1 handful (6 ounces/170 g) dry uncooked noodles of choice (see Note)

1 tablespoon green onion, thinly sliced

1 small (225 g) Persian cucumber, skin on, thinly sliced

¼ cup (25 g) grated red cabbage

½ medium carrot, cut into matchsticks

2 cilantro sprigs, leaves picked off

2 tablespoons fresh mint leaves, finely chopped

2 tablespoons lime juice

In a small bowl, combine peanut butter, soy sauce, sesame oil, cane sugar, and 1 tablespoon water and mix together until smooth.

In a medium pot over medium-high heat, bring 2 quarts (2 L) water to a boil. Add noodles and cook according to package instructions. Strain noodles and place in a large bowl.

Combine with peanut butter sauce mixture.

Sprinkle in green onion, cucumber, red cabbage, carrot, cilantro, mint, and lime juice.

Note: Consider using kelp noodles, spiralized zucchini noodles, heart of palm noodles, or shirataki noodles.

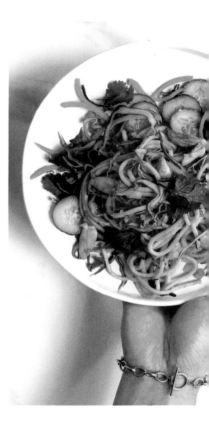

Serves 2

I trust my intuition.

PROTEINS

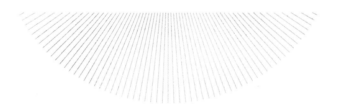

Grandma's Fried Rice

My maternal and paternal grandmothers would make their own version of fried rice for special occasions. This is a terrifically quick and easy one-bowl meal with everything you need—protein, carbohydrates, and veggies. It can be eaten on its own or served as a side dish. Throw some leftover rice in a pan and see what ingredients you have on hand; fried rice is often made with whatever you have left in the fridge. Spinach and sausage are some of my favorite add-ins, but the sky's the limit! Allow the rice to crisp up on its edges for extra crunch and finish with a dollop of ketchup.

¾ cup (160 g) cooked short-grain white rice (see Note)

2 eggs

½ teaspoon cane sugar

1 tablespoon avocado oil

¼ cup (30 g) peeled, roughly chopped white onion

¼ teaspoon sea salt

1 (¼-inch/6 mm) knob fresh ginger, peeled, grated or minced

1 (3¼-ounce/92 g) sausage (vegan or meat), sliced into coins, or 2 slices bacon, chopped

1 green onion, white and green parts separated, finely chopped

OPTIONAL
2 tablespoons ketchup

Make sure your rice is not wet and mushy. The best way to prevent this is to leave cooked rice in the fridge overnight. Once the rice is nice and dry, whisk together the eggs and sugar and mix into the rice, coating each grain. Set aside.

Heat a large nonstick pan over medium-high, then add oil and warm for a few seconds. Add onion, salt, ginger, and sausage. Turn the heat down to medium and cook until lightly browned. Scoop out sausage, onion, and ginger and discard any excessive oil if needed, leaving about 1 tablespoon oil in the pan for the rice.

Add the egg and rice mixture to the pan. Stir-fry continuously for 2 minutes by shaking the pan and moving the ingredients around. Add the white part of the green onion and cook for another 2 minutes, then stir in ketchup (if using).

Stir in the green part of the green onion and serve the fried rice immediately.

Note: If your days tend to get very busy, stock up on a few pouches of precooked rice, which is commonly found in a grocer's freezer section. One 10-ounce pouch will work for this recipe. Cook according to the instructions found on the package a day before using and leave the rice uncovered in the fridge to dry out.

PROTEINS

Serves 2

I am open to receiving good thoughts, words, and love.

Shiitake Chicken Noodle Bowl

If you suddenly get the urge to slurp down a big bowl of yummy noodles during your pregnancy, you're not alone! It happens to many people, and it's a sign from your body that it's using lots of energy to build your baby. This dish, which balances well-portioned carbohydrates (noodles) with protein (chicken) and fat (in the chicken thighs), is a great way to meet that need. Shiitake mushrooms, red cabbage, ginger, garlic, and black vinegar (prized for its high antioxidant count and thicker texture, similar to balsamic vinegar) round out the nutritional benefits for a complete healthy "noodle bar" meal that is as good as any street food I've enjoyed!

CHICKEN MARINADE

3 tablespoons rice vinegar

2 tablespoons soy sauce (substitution: Bragg Liquid Aminos or gluten-free tamari)

2 tablespoons peeled and grated ginger

1 garlic clove, grated

NOODLE SAUCE

2 tablespoons soy sauce (substitution: Bragg Liquid Aminos or gluten-free tamari)

1 tablespoon sesame oil

2 tablespoons black vinegar (substitution: rice vinegar, balsamic vinegar, apple cider vinegar)

1 teaspoon cane sugar

————

2 chicken thighs, boneless, skin on

4 dried (40 g) or 4 fresh (20 g) shiitake mushrooms, thinly sliced

Combine the ingredients for the marinade and pour it over the chicken thighs. Cover and refrigerate for an hour.

Combine ingredients for the noodle sauce and set aside.

If using dried shiitakes, rinse and soak them in water at room temperature for an hour while the chicken is marinating.

Heat a large pan over medium-high. Add 2 tablespoons avocado oil and warm for a few seconds. Add red cabbage in a single layer and lightly brown for 10 minutes. Add maple syrup and cook for another 2 minutes. Remove from the pan and set aside.

In the same pan, add 2 tablespoons avocado oil, brown the white onion for 7 to 10 minutes, then add shiitake mushrooms, adding more oil if needed. Cook for 5 to 7 minutes, transfer from the pan to a small bowl, and set aside.

Add the remaining 2 tablespoons avocado oil to the pan. Place the chicken (skin side down) in the pan, pour the marinade over the chicken, and cook over medium heat for 5 minutes, until browned. Turn the chicken over and cook for 5 to 7 minutes, until cooked through. Remove from the pan, cut into thin slices, and top with the juices from the pan. Set aside.

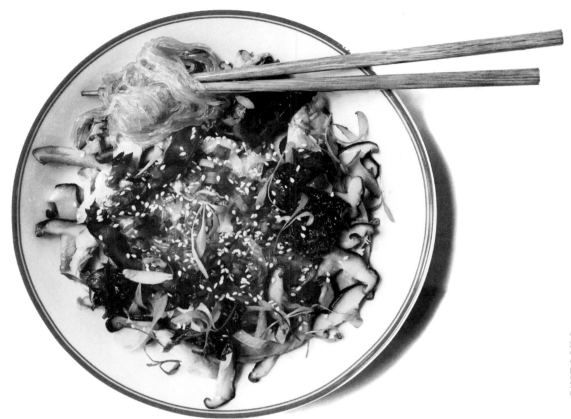

PROTEINS

6 tablespoons (90 ml) avocado oil, plus more as needed

1 cup (95 g) red cabbage, thinly grated

1 tablespoon maple syrup

¼ white onion (30 g), peeled, thinly sliced

1 handful (6 ounces/170 g) dry uncooked noodles of choice (see Note, page 201)

1 green onion, finely chopped

In a medium pot over medium-high heat, bring 2 quarts (2 L) water to a boil. Add the noodles and cook according to package instructions, then strain.

In a large bowl, combine noodles, noodle sauce, red cabbage, white onion and mushrooms, and chicken. Garnish with green onion. Enjoy warm.

Serves 2

I welcome change.

Garlic–Butter Steak Bites

When you get a craving for steak during pregnancy, this is a perfect way to enjoy it. Cubed into bite-size chunks, you can use it in a nourishing bowl, customized as you like with vegetables or grains of your choice. The buttery garlic flavor with a hint of rosemary makes it delectably tasty, and it's a cinch to prepare! It also stores well for a few days, so consider making double to help quickly make lunch or dinner later in the week. Try making a bowl of steak bites with Garlic Broccoli Rabe (page 196), Cauliflower Millet Mash (page 198), and a scoop of sauerkraut to make a super nourishing meal in minutes.

¾ teaspoon sea salt

½ teaspoon black pepper

1 pound (455 g) rib-eye steak, boneless, cut into 1-inch (2.5 cm) cubes

6 tablespoons (85 g) butter, plus more for searing (substitution: vegan butter—I recommend Miyoko's Creamery)

2 garlic cloves, finely minced

1 tablespoon fresh rosemary, finely minced

Salt and pepper all sides of the steak and set aside.

In a large ceramic or stainless-steel pan over medium-high heat, melt the butter. Add garlic and rosemary and lightly brown for 20 seconds.

Flash-cook the steak flat in the pan, without stacking the meat, for 3 to 4 minutes each side to brown the edges.

Plate the steak, drizzle with the rosemary and garlic butter sauce, and serve hot.

Serves 2

My healing starts today.

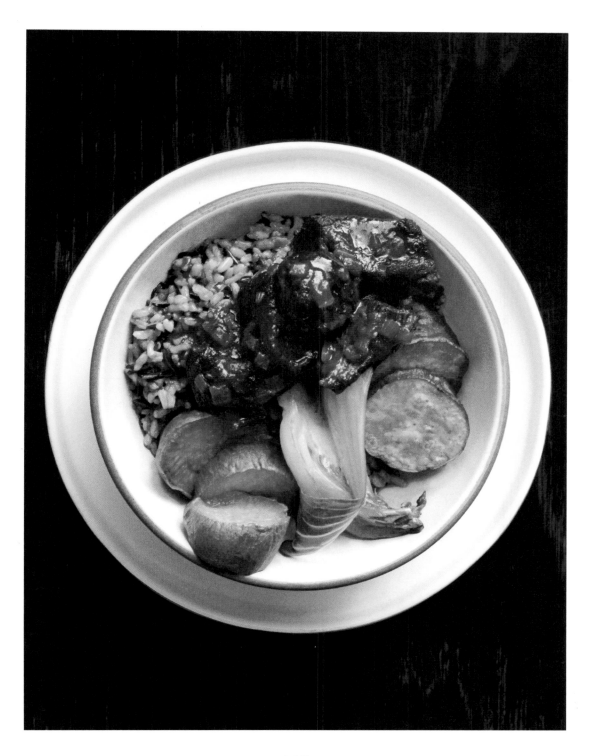

Roasted Lemony Chicken

I used to make this dish in the United Kingdom when I was pregnant with my daughter Khefri. I vividly recall the whole chickens I bought at the butcher's—smaller and leaner than their American counterparts after being raised in pastures eating bugs and pecking in mineral-rich soil. My mouth waters just thinking about their flavor merging with lemons, capers, and small, in-season tomatoes—food is memory, after all, and each wonderful meal can hold part of the story of your life. The sauce will be thickened with gelatin from the bone-in thighs—an added boon in pregnancy. Make this satisfying dish on a Sunday so it's ready to go for an easy weeknight meal. Serve it with Cauliflower Millet Mash (page 198) to soak up the fragrant juices.

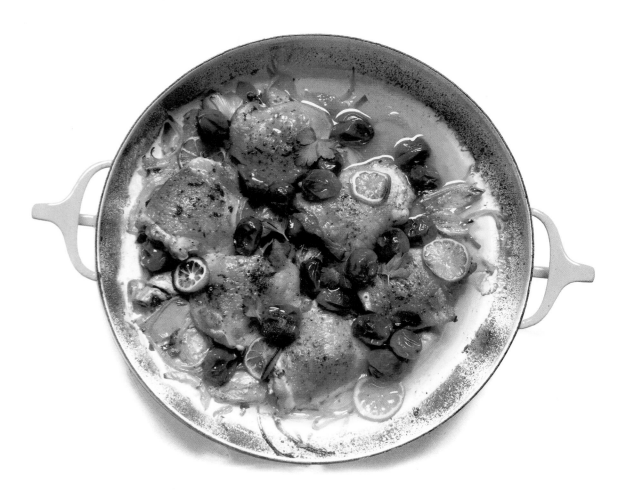

2 lemons

4 tablespoons (60 ml) avocado oil, plus more as needed

2 tablespoons capers

½ cup (90 g) green olives, unpitted

1 (14-ounce/400 g) can artichoke hearts in water, strained, rinsed

1 (120 g) white onion, peeled, halved, thinly sliced

2 garlic cloves, roughly chopped

2 teaspoons parsley, roughly chopped

2 tablespoons black mustard seed, smashed with a rolling pin

2 teaspoons sea salt, plus more as needed

1 teaspoon black pepper

6 bone-in, skin-on chicken thighs (1¾ pounds/750 g total), rinsed, patted dry

1 cup (240 ml) stock of choice

2 cups (290 g) small cherry tomatoes

Preheat the oven to 425°F (220°C).

In a large cast-iron skillet, braising pan, or 3-quart baking dish, combine the juice of 1 lemon, 2 tablespoons oil, capers, olives, artichoke hearts, onion, garlic, and parsley. Make sure ingredients lie flat.

In a small bowl, combine mustard seed, salt, pepper, and remaining 2 tablespoons oil, then rub all over the chicken.

Slice the second lemon, skin on, into 6 rounds and set aside.

Arrange the chicken (skin side up) in a single layer on top of the artichoke mixture and cover with the lemon slices. Place skillet on the top rack of the oven and cook for 20 minutes (set a timer). After 20 minutes, add the stock.

On a separate parchment–lined roasting pan, coat the tomatoes with oil and a dash of salt. Place the pan in the oven with the chicken, on the bottom rack. Roast for 20 minutes (set a timer) or until tomatoes are lightly caramelized. Remove tomatoes from the oven and set aside.

Continue to roast the chicken for another 30 minutes or until the chicken skin is golden brown. Remove skillet from the oven, add caramelized tomatoes and any juices to the chicken, and serve.

PROTEINS

Serves 2 to 3

I am human and I am making a difference in the world.

Coconut Apple Liver Pâté

Liver is one of those pregnancy power foods many people intend to consume, but don't always pull off. Maybe it's because modern humans have lost the habit of consuming it regularly and therefore never developed the taste for it. Beef liver is the most nutrient-dense (and intense-tasting) type of all, but if you need a gentler entry to the liver world, try this pâté instead. I've taken mild-tasting chicken liver and combined it with sweet apple and neutral coconut cream to make it super palatable. This is great as an afternoon snack with crackers and is quite easy to make once you get the hang of it. Try to consume a few ounces of liver weekly—a small portion goes a long way to delivering the nutrients your baby needs to develop! You can store this pâté in a glass jar for up to a week in the fridge.

2 tablespoons ghee or unsalted butter

½ teaspoon sea salt

1 (120 g) white onion, roughly chopped

1 (130 g) apple, peeled, de-seeded, and cut into ¼-inch (6 mm) cubes

1 teaspoon ground nutmeg

½ cup (120 ml) cold water

½ pound (225 g) chicken liver, rinsed, roughly chopped

1 (5.4-ounce/160 ml) can coconut cream

Heat a large pan over medium-high, then add the ghee, salt, and onion. Cook until lightly browned, about 7 minutes. Add the apple, nutmeg, and cold water, reduce the heat to medium-low, and cook partially covered for 10 minutes, until apples are soft.

Add chopped chicken liver, return the heat to medium-high, and cook for 10 minutes, uncovered.

Add the coconut cream and cook for another 10 minutes, stirring regularly. Cook down the liquid if needed to make sure the mixture is moist, but not too wet.

Place the mixture in a food processor and blend until smooth. Enjoy warm, or cool before storing in a glass container in the fridge.

Serves 2

Everything in my body is working to help my baby develop healthily.

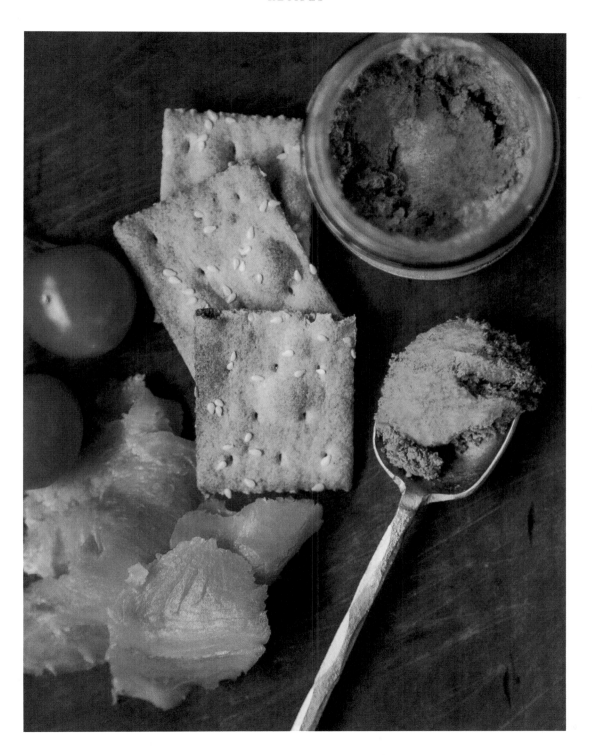

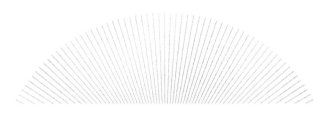

BREAKFAST

Agni Stewed Apples & Prunes

I love giving my digestion a gentle start in the morning, and stewed fruits are a wonderful way to do that—they're hydrating, sweet, and full of fiber to ensure everything keeps moving. Add this warming compote to some Millet Ginger Congee (page 182) for a delicious breakfast that will help feed the fire (called "agni" in Ayurveda) of digestion early in the day, allowing it to build up naturally without overwhelming it first thing. For a good morning ritual, start by drinking a glass of water, taking your prenatal supplements, then following with this breakfast or, if you're not yet ready to eat, with a fresh juice (see page 240). Note: This isn't high in protein, so a midmorning protein-rich snack is wise.

1 (110 g) apple, peeled, de-seeded, and cut into ¼-inch (6 mm) cubes

7 prunes, pitted

¼ teaspoon ground cinnamon

1 clove

¼ teaspoon ground cardamom

2 cups (480 ml) cold water

1 tablespoon butter or ghee

In a small saucepan, combine apples, prunes, cinnamon, clove, cardamom, and cold water. Cook, partially covered, for 1 hour over medium-low heat.

Turn off heat and stir in ghee.

Eat warm and drink the extra liquid to support your digestion and elimination.

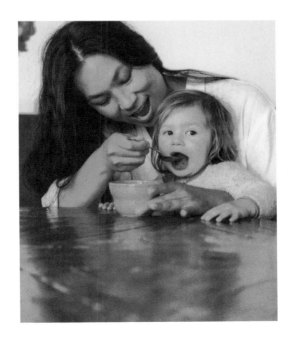

Serves 2

I am grateful for the food I am about to eat. My baby is grateful too.

Cardamom Breakfast Bowl

This grain-free bowl of soaked nuts and seeds will keep your belly full for hours. A little goes a long way! It's like a soft granola, chewy and nutty and best topped with fresh fruit, milk, yogurt, or kefir. It takes just five minutes to prepare the night before, giving you a quick and hearty meal for the morning. Perhaps breakfast in bed?

½ cup (54 g) slivered almonds

½ cup (55 g) chopped walnuts

¼ cup (30 g) pumpkin seeds

2 Medjool dates (50 g), pitted

2 tablespoons hemp seeds

2 tablespoons chia seeds

pinch of sea salt

2 cups (475 ml) cold water

½ cup (120 ml) milk of choice (almond, coconut, cow, macadamia, oat, rice, or goat), plus more for serving

1 teaspoon vanilla extract

1 teaspoon ground cardamom

TOPPING OPTIONS
fresh berries, apricots, peaches, ground cinnamon

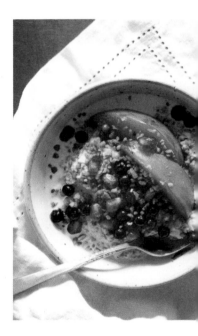

In a food processor, coarsely chop or pulse almonds, walnuts, pumpkin seeds, and dates. Empty processor contents into a large bowl.

Mix in hemp, chia seeds, and salt. Add cold water, cover, and refrigerate overnight.

The next morning, strain the mixture through a fine sieve and return contents to the same bowl (rinse bowl if needed). Add milk of choice, vanilla extract, and ground cardamom, then stir. Let it sit for ½ hour.

Enjoy hot or at room temperature with a splash of milk and layers of your favorite toppings.

Serves 2 or 3

I am curious, open, and vulnerable.

Blueberry Cottage Cheese Crepe

Keeping a stash of blueberries (wild ones, if possible!) in the freezer is a smart move; you'll have them on hand for these delicious crepes, as well as other mixed-berry compotes and smoothies. Thanks to their high fiber and polyphenol count, blueberries are a great prebiotic food, meaning they feed the health-promoting probiotic bacteria in your GI tract. And when your gut microbiome thrives, this ripples over to support your baby's microbiome and the immune system that functions in close relationship with it. (During a vaginal delivery, a baby gets their first dose of gut flora from their mother.) Eating plenty of prebiotic-rich fruits and green vegetables during pregnancy can give your baby a head start on great gut and immune health!

WILD BLUEBERRY COMPOTE

4 cups (560 g) fresh or frozen wild blueberries

¼ cup (60 ml) lemon juice

½ cup (100 g) cane sugar

½ cup (120 ml) cold water

———————

1 cup (225 g) cottage cheese (see Note)

4 medium eggs (see Note)

½ teaspoon vanilla extract

¼ teaspoon sea salt

1 dash ground cardamom

1 tablespoon butter (substitution: vegan butter—I recommend Miyoko's Creamery)

In a small saucepan over medium-high heat, combine the blueberries, lemon juice, sugar, and cold water and cook for 5 to 7 minutes. Mash the berries with a fork, then cook for another 15 minutes until large bubbles appear. With a firm rubber spatula, scrape the compote into a bowl and set aside to cool.

In a medium bowl, whisk together the cottage cheese, eggs, vanilla extract, salt, and cardamom to make the crepe batter.

In a large nonstick pan over medium heat, melt the butter. Pour ½ cup (120 ml) crepe batter into the pan. Once bubbles begin to appear, reduce heat to medium-low and cook for an additional 4 minutes until light golden on the bottom, then flip and cook to golden on the other side. Set aside on a plate, then gently roll it up. Watch your fingers! Repeat with the remaining batter.

Scoop blueberry compote over crepe and serve warm.

Note: For cottage cheese, I recommend the organic, pasture-raised brand Good Culture, which contains live, active probiotic cultures to support gut health. For eggs, I like purchasing from organic pasture-raised Vital Farms, which also produces ghee and butter. Blueberry compote can be enjoyed hot or cold. Refrigerate any leftover compote in a jar for up to 2 weeks.

BREAKFAST

Serves 4

I take this moment to connect with my food, my body, and my baby.

Silky Egg Custard

This is another way for pregnant moms to eat their eggs as a quick snack. You can easily steam this for a few minutes, add a little sauce, and spoon it up. The texture is soft and neutral, as though you are eating a savory pudding. This is a traditional Chinese dish, which might take some patience to master, but no matter how you create it, you get a healthy dose of choline to support your baby's brain development. One egg yolk contains about 35 percent of your daily requirement.

3 eggs

¼ teaspoon sea salt

1¼ cups (300 ml) warm water, plus more for steaming

TOPPINGS
1 teaspoon sesame oil

1 teaspoon soy sauce (substitution: Bragg Liquid Aminos or gluten-free tamari)

½ green onion, thinly sliced

In a steamer over medium-high heat, bring 1 inch (2.5 cm) water to a boil. Once the water boils, reduce heat to medium-low.

You will need two bowls: one to mix the eggs, salt, and water in, and another (preferably wide, short, and heatproof for even cooking, like a soup bowl) that fits in the steamer.

In the first bowl, whisk eggs well with a fork or chopsticks until the mixture is very smooth. Add salt, stir in warm water, and give it another good stir.

Using a sieve, strain egg mixture into the second bowl, which will be going in the steamer. If there are any bubbles, remove with a spoon. This process will result in a smooth custard texture.

Gently place the bowl in the steamer and cover the bowl with a plate light enough so that steam can get in and stay in, without being blocked out completely. Then, place the lid on the steamer and steam for 10 minutes over medium-low heat (set a timer). Turn off the heat and let it steam for another 5 minutes (again, set a timer). You are looking for a soft jelly-like jiggle with the egg cooked all the way through.

Remove the bowl using kitchen towels or oven mitts and let it rest for 2 minutes. Cut slits across the top into squares to allow the sauce to sink in.

Top with oil, soy sauce, and green onion. Serve hot.

Serves 2 to 4

I cherish my body and how it is nourishing my baby and m.

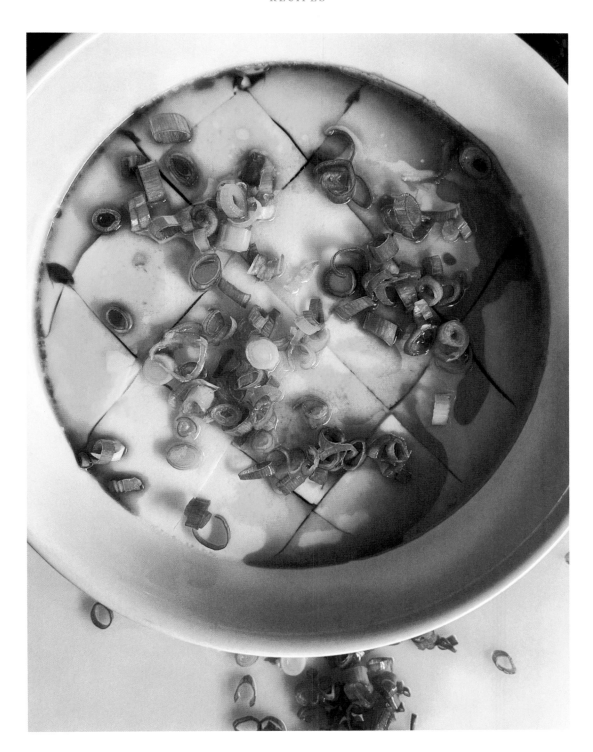

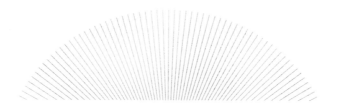

SMOOTHIES

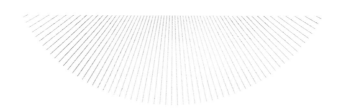

Refreshing Papaya Smoothie

Pregnancy and heartburn can go hand in hand, especially around the third trimester when the stomach can get cramped by the growing uterus. Many pregnant women find that fresh papaya helps soothe this irritation, while also supporting healthy elimination. Here, it is made into a delectable smoothie enlivened with lime juice and a pinch of salt. You can trust you are giving your body (and your baby) a real treat as you sip on it—ripe papaya is loaded with beta-carotene (the precursor to vitamin A) and vitamin C, along with calcium, magnesium, potassium, folate, and lots of gut-supportive fiber.

1 small ripe orange papaya, de-seeded, scooped

1 cup (240 ml) water or unsweetened milk (almond, macadamia, coconut, rice, oat)

1 teaspoon honey

1 teaspoon lime juice

pinch of sea salt

OPTIONAL
serving of your favorite protein powder and/or collagen powder, plus an extra splash of water or milk

Blend all ingredients in a high-speed blender to desired consistency and enjoy right away.

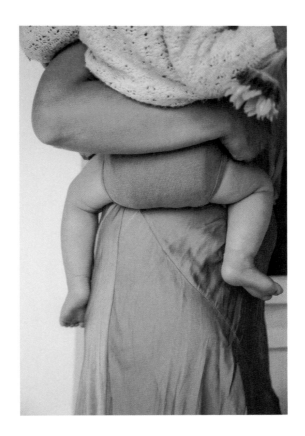

Serves 1

I thrive. My baby thrives.

Black Sesame Coconut Smoothie

A former client who spent time in Hawaii taught me this smoothie recipe, which I have made for many years now as a satiating breakfast or hearty snack. This smoothie is as filling, creamy, and tasty as a milkshake! Though you can use frozen coconut meat and boxed coconut water, give it a whirl using a fresh coconut if that is available—the effort to hack off the top is well rewarded as you reveal one of nature's finest sources of electrolytes, good fats, and fiber. Black sesame seeds are becoming easier to find these days; these are used regularly in Chinese cuisine, especially for desserts. They contain calcium, iron, magnesium, and lots of antioxidants to support your baby's development and health in utero. You do need a lot of the seeds to get the benefits, so let this recipe introduce you to black sesame, and then turn to my other recipes in *The First Forty Days* for more ways to use it!

1½ cups (360 ml) total coconut water and meat (equal amounts of each; fresh, if available)

2 teaspoons black sesame seeds

¼ cup (35 g) macadamia nuts, unsalted

½ teaspoon organic vanilla extract

pinch of ground cinnamon

OPTIONAL
serving of your favorite protein powder and/or collagen powder, plus an extra splash of coconut water

Blend all ingredients in a high-speed blender to desired consistency and enjoy right away.

Serves 1

I am enough. I am supported. I am loved.

Cacao Avocado Spirulina Smoothie

I love the convenience of a nutrient-packed smoothie. At home, I'll use whatever I have on hand, blending fruits and nut butters or avocado with some coconut water into a hearty, on-the-go meal or snack. A smoothie is a safe space to experiment; add a little more of this, a little less of that, and see what flavors and textures light you up. This smoothie is filling and just sweet enough, and the bright blue-green from the spirulina makes it fun to drink. Spirulina is a super algae containing chlorophyll, which supports your blood cells by transporting oxygen throughout the body.

1½ cups (360 ml) unsweetened milk of choice (almond, macadamia, coconut, rice, oat)

2 Medjool dates, pitted

½ medium avocado, pitted

1 tablespoon cacao powder

1 teaspoon spirulina powder (see Note)

¼ teaspoon vanilla extract

OPTIONAL
serving of your favorite protein powder and/or collagen powder, plus an extra splash of milk

Blend all ingredients in a high-speed blender to desired consistency and enjoy right away.

Note: You can commonly find spirulina powder at your local health food store. We prefer the Pure Hawaiian Spirulina brand.

Serves 1

I am courageous.

Wild Blueberry Nut Butter Smoothie

There is something comforting about a good ol' peanut butter and jelly sandwich, and now this childhood favorite takes the form of a delectable smoothie. Wild blueberries join the crunch of cacao and the healthy fat in your favorite nut butter to create a delicious meal that satisfies and uplifts. This smoothie packs a hydrating punch too. It's easy enough to become dehydrated when you're not pregnant—and much more so when you are!

1 cup (240 ml) unsweetened milk of choice (almond, macadamia, coconut, rice, oat)

2 Medjool dates, pitted

1 banana

½ cup (95 g) fresh or frozen wild blueberries

¼ avocado, pitted

2 tablespoons (30 g) nut butter of choice

1 teaspoon raw cacao nibs

1 teaspoon chia seeds

OPTIONAL
serving of your favorite protein powder and/or collagen powder, plus an extra splash of milk

Blend all ingredients in a high-speed blender to desired consistency and enjoy right away.

Serves 1

I am beautiful inside and out.

Dragon Fruit Smoothie

The exotic dragon fruit (pitaya) is a beauty inside and out—and it's got an equally impressive nutritional profile. When you push past the soft, spiky, hot-pink rind and dig into the mildly sweet and tart, black seed–speckled flesh, you take in vitamin C, calcium, protein, iron, and potassium. Dragon fruit can be elusive, but today it's becoming easier to find at specialty markets, or in the frozen food aisle. If you can't locate any near you, coconut meat from a young coconut makes an excellent substitute.

1 fresh or 2 frozen pouches
(200 g total) dragon fruit

½ cup (80 g) fresh or frozen
wild blueberries

2 Medjool dates, pitted

1 cup (240 ml) unsweetened
milk of choice (almond,
macadamia, coconut,
rice, oat)

OPTIONAL
serving of your favorite
protein powder and/or
collagen powder, plus an
extra splash of milk

Blend all ingredients in a high-speed blender to desired consistency and enjoy right away.

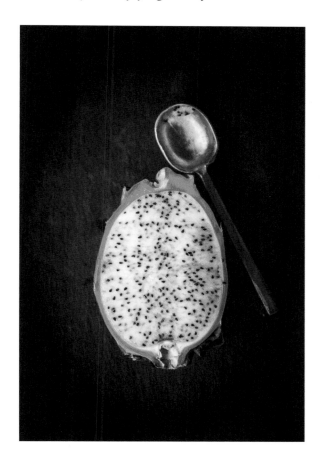

Serves 1

My mind, heart, and body are connected.

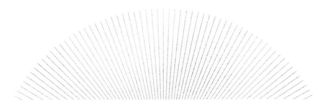

SWEETS

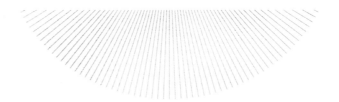

Rujak (Indonesian Fruit Dip)

Robin Lim, a master midwife and one of our treasured wise ones, encourages the moms-to-be in her bustling Bali clinic to snack on rujak during their pregnancies. A favorite of Indonesian grandmothers, this pungent dip hits all the bases: sweet, salty, and sour. And when paired the traditional way with fresh fruits, it delivers vitamins, fiber, and hydration. In Indonesia, rujak is used to soothe nausea in pregnant women and is best enjoyed with friends and family, sitting around the kitchen table, dipping, talking, eating, and laughing.

DIPPING SAUCE

2 tablespoons tamarind paste (found online or in Asian markets)

1 teaspoon coconut sugar or brown sugar, plus more to taste

¼ cup (60 ml) filtered water, plus more as needed

FRUIT AND VEGETABLE OPTIONS

green mango, peeled, cut into matchsticks

jicama, peeled, cut into matchsticks

apple, peeled, sliced

cucumber, peeled, sliced

pear, peeled, sliced

Combine tamarind paste, coconut or brown sugar, and filtered water in a small bowl, adding more water if needed until a thick, slightly runny texture is reached. Add more sugar if needed, as the tamarind is naturally tart.

Cut your fruits and veggies of choice to dip in the sauce and enjoy!

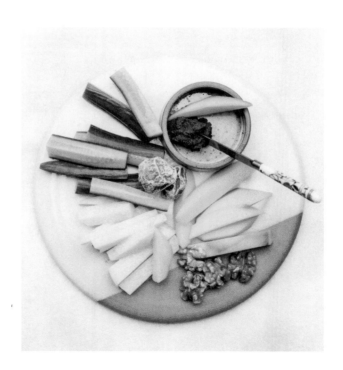

SWEETS

Serves 2

I trust my body. I trust my birth process.

Cacao Chia Pudding

Sometimes a simple treat is all you need to change your mood and perspective. For me, this shift often comes from chocolate. This decadent-tasting pudding is easy to prepare—and deceptively nutritious. The pudding gets its body from chia seeds, which plump up when soaked and are rich in fiber, antioxidants, and omega-3s. Once you've mastered this recipe, you'll always want it on hand so you can dip a spoon in for a quick hit of joy.

1 cup (170 g) chia seeds

½ teaspoon cinnamon powder

2 teaspoons unsweetened cacao powder

½ teaspoon vanilla extract

pinch of sea salt

2 cups (480 ml) unsweetened milk of choice (almond, cow, macadamia, coconut, rice, oat), plus more as needed

1 tablespoon maple syrup

TOPPING SUGGESTIONS
apple slices, berries, stone fruit slices, walnuts, coconut flakes

In a mixing bowl, mix chia seeds, cinnamon powder, cacao powder, vanilla extract, salt, and milk. Whisk well. Once the pudding is thick from the expansion of the chia seeds, roughly an hour, add maple syrup and whisk some more. If the pudding is too thick, stir in some more milk. Add toppings and serve.

Note: You can place all ingredients except the fruits into a 16-ounce (480 ml) glass Mason jar, whisk away, then store in the fridge. The next day, you can add fruits and eat from the jar.

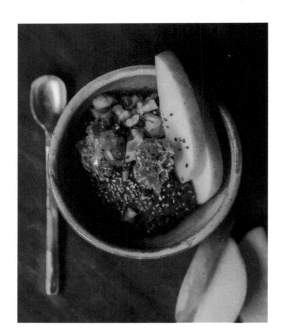

Serves 4

I am present in my body, feeling my feet, taking a deep long breath.

India's Chocolate Delights

India, my second daughter, is a joy to mother and to cook with. Sandwiched in age between her elder sister, Khefri, and younger brother, Jude, India has a love for—and a real gift for—the art of cooking. Pescatarian meals and baked goods have become her areas of specialty, and I willingly let her lead! India first made these chocolate cookie treats to ensure that our kitchen was always stocked with healthy indulgences and so we always have access to a quick bite during our busy weekdays. They are gluten-free, egg-free, and totally scrumptious. If a teenager loves making them, I can pretty much guarantee that you will too. If you want to turn them into a higher-protein, more satiating snack, smother some nut butter on top. No need to refrigerate them because they won't last long! If you like, you can use one of the alternative sweeteners listed in the Pantry section (page 169).

⅓ cup (75 ml) coconut oil, solidified in the fridge or on the counter overnight (see Tip)

½ cup (112 g) coconut sugar

2 teaspoons vanilla extract

2 tablespoons almond milk

1 cup (96 g) almond flour

1 cup (125 g) oat flour

½ teaspoon baking soda

½ teaspoon baking powder

¼ teaspoon sea salt

½ cup (85 g) dark chocolate chips (I like Hu Kitchen Snacking & Baking Dark Chocolate Gems)

Preheat the oven to 350°F (177°C). Line a baking sheet with parchment paper.

In the bowl of a stand mixer with a paddle attachment (or using a mixing bowl and a spoon), combine coconut oil and coconut sugar. Mix on high for 1 minute, then add vanilla extract and milk. Continue to mix for another 30 seconds.

With the mixer running, add the almond flour and mix for 10 seconds. Add the oat flour, baking soda, baking powder, and salt. Continue to mix for about 20 seconds, scraping down the sides and bottom of the bowl with a spatula, until a large dough ball forms. Turn off mixer and stir in the chocolate chips with a spatula.

Using a ½-inch (12 mm) wide cookie scooper or a spoon, scoop out about 1½ tablespoons of dough at a time. Arrange on the prepared baking sheet, with about 2 inches (5 cm) space in between them. Bake in the oven for 12 minutes, until edges are lightly golden. Remember to set a timer.

Remove from the oven and let the tray rest for 10 minutes on the counter, then eat warm and enjoy!

Tip: If your coconut oil is solid to start, for easier measuring, melt a small amount in a small pan over low heat, then measure out ⅓ cup (75 ml).

Makes 8 cookies

My child and I are discovering the world together.

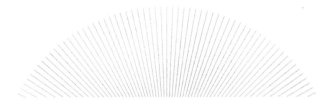

TEAS, TONICS
& ELIXIRS

At MotherBees, we pride ourselves on sourcing unusual ingredients from cultures around the world. We love how each ingredient offers a different health benefit while giving us a window into the grower's passion and motivation. In this Teas, Tonics & Elixirs section, I highlight some of the more exotic ingredients in the MotherBees pantry, though they should be fairly easy to source. The recipes themselves are simple, showcasing just one or two key ingredients—a special herb, or a lesser known fruit. Each ingredient is chosen for its gentle, healing effects; all are safe for use during pregnancy as directed in the recipes, in moderation. If you stumble upon something unfamiliar, I encourage you to stay curious and give it a chance. You may discover a new ally to accompany you along your pregnancy journey.

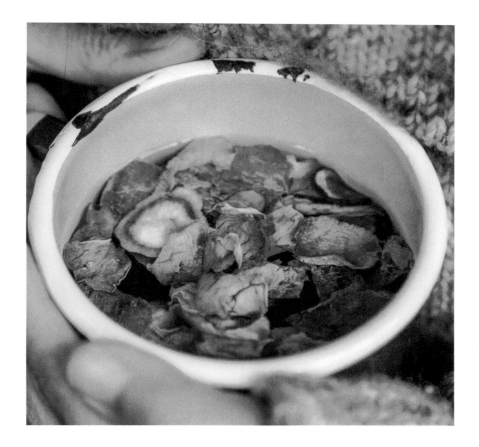

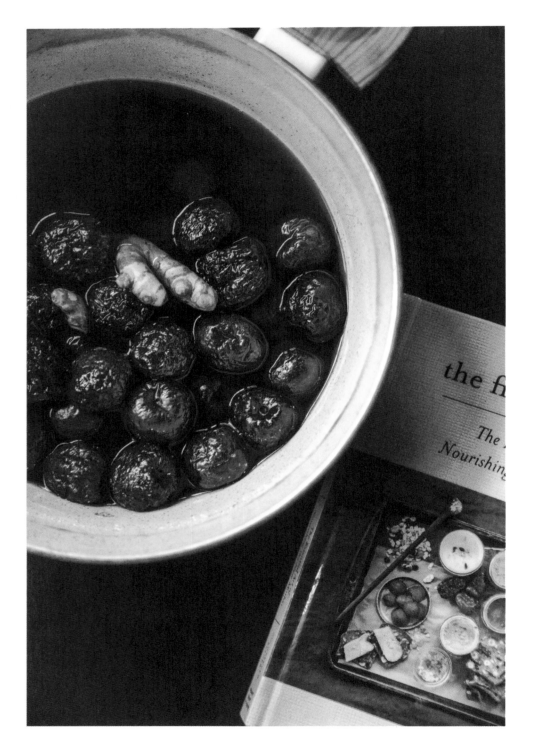

Warming Jujube Tea

At MotherBees, we are huge fans of jujubes. These small stone fruits, also known as red dates, have long been prized in China for their high levels of antioxidants, vitamin C, and minerals that can help with sleep, skin, circulation, and more. When I found my source of organic jujubes, Farmer David in Southern California, I fell further in love with this fruit. At David's farm, you can eat the fresh fruits off the trees, but since the growing season is short, the most common way to use them is dried, then cooked in teas, broths, and soups, offering a mildly sweet, slightly caramelly note.

3 dry jujubes, rinsed, pitted

1 (½-inch/12 mm) knob fresh ginger, skin on, cut in half

1 tablespoon raisins

½ teaspoon cinnamon powder

½ teaspoon dark brown sugar

2 cups (480 ml) cold water

In a small pot, combine all ingredients and cook over medium heat for 15 minutes.

Strain the tea, mashing the jujubes with a spoon to squeeze out all the extra liquid so no tea is wasted. Discard jujubes.

Enjoy the tea warm!

Note: You may notice a white foam when boiling jujubes for tea. This is normal; simply skim it off before drinking.

TEAS, TONICS & ELIXIRS

Serves 1; best for third trimester

My foundation is built on positive thoughts and words.

Jujube & Adzuki Tea

Adzuki beans are a nutrient-dense food that supports energy levels while providing a good source of protein and complex carbohydrates. These mild beans are also rich in antioxidants and can aid the growth and repair of cells for mom and baby. In Asian cultures, jujubes and adzuki beans are used to support a mother's milk and overall postpartum health. Here, I've paired the two in a pretty pink tea with a light, sweet flavor. A touch of kombu seaweed adds a subtle umami flavor while delivering iodine, an important nutrient for pregnant and breastfeeding women. Feel free to eat the cooked adzuki beans to consume more fiber.

6 cups (1.4 L) cold water

3 dry jujubes, rinsed, pitted

1 (15-ounce/425 g) can adzuki beans, strained, rinsed

1 (3-inch/7.5 cm) strip dry kombu seaweed

1 (1-inch/2.5 cm) knob fresh ginger, skin on, sliced

pinch of sea salt

2 tablespoons honey

In a small pot over medium heat, bring cold water to a soft boil. Add dry jujubes, adzuki beans, kombu, ginger, and pinch of salt. Reduce the heat to low and cook for 2 hours. (See Note on page 231.)

Turn off heat, strain, add honey, and sip warm.

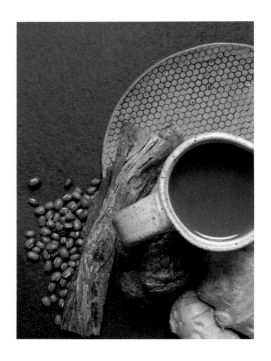

Makes 3 to 4 cups (720 to 960 ml); best for third trimester

I take care of my bountiful body.

Asian Pear Ginger Tea

Asian pears are super crunchy with a fresh, lightly sweet flavor. In Chinese medicine, the fruit is used to reduce excess mucus, calming and nourishing the Lungs, the organs where we hold sadness or grief in the body. When Lung chi is healthy, we can think clearly and are open to new ideas, providing a strong foundation for our growing baby. I love the subtle taste of Asian pear as it cooks down and mingles with jujube and ginger, but I always save a raw pear to munch on throughout the day.

2 quarts (2 L) cold water

3 dry jujubes, rinsed, pitted

1 Asian pear, washed, peeled, de-seeded, sliced

1 (1-inch/2.5 cm) knob fresh ginger, skin on, washed, sliced

In a medium pot over medium-high heat, add cold water, jujubes, Asian pear, and ginger and cook, partially covered, for 30 minutes. Turn down heat to medium-low and cook for another 2 hours. (See Note on page 231.)

Turn off heat, strain, drink the tea, and enjoy the cooked pear slices on the side.

TEAS, TONICS & ELIXIRS

Serves 2; best for second and third trimesters

I am grateful I am pregnant.

Snow Ear & Lotus Seeds Tonic

Snow ear has been used for centuries as a tonic in late pregnancy, helping maintain the skin's elasticity as your belly and breasts stretch and grow, increasing the elasticity of the perineum to prepare for birth, and helping give babies smooth skin. Also known as snow fungus, white fungus, or white wood ear, this special ingredient can be found in most Chinese grocery stores or online. Lotus seeds come from the stunning lotus flower, a symbol of enlightenment and rebirth, and they are considered a superfood for pregnant women, tonifying the Spleen and Kidneys to help support energy or chi. When made with water, this beverage will be lightly sweet; for more flavor, use Asian Pear Ginger Tea (page 233).

1 (20 g) dry snow ear fungus (see Notes)

6 cups (1.4 L) cold water or Asian Pear Ginger Tea (page 233)

2 tablespoons lotus seeds, washed

1 egg, whisked

1 tablespoon honey (omit if using Asian Pear Ginger Tea)

In a medium bowl, combine snow ear and enough water to entirely cover and let soak for 20 minutes, until completely softened.

Discard the soaking water and rinse snow ear under fresh water. Cut out the slightly dark yellow center and discard, then chop snow ear into small bite-size pieces.

In a medium pot, combine cold water or tea, snow ear, and lotus seeds and cook over medium-high heat until boiling. Turn down the heat to medium-low and cook for 2 hours until the snow ear is soft and gelatinous, and the lotus seeds are soft. Add more water if needed.

Turn the heat back to medium-high and wait until the temperature and bubbles rise. Stir in the whisked egg and cook for 2 minutes.

Turn off the heat and stir in honey (if using) when ready to drink the tonic; the softened snow ear and lotus seeds can be eaten.

Notes: When cooked down, snow ear fungus should have a slippery and gelatinous texture. When shopping, make sure you choose a more yellow-tinted, rather than white, snow ear fungus.

Eating the softened snow ear and lotus seeds is part of this tonic experience—enjoy the different textures in your cup!

Serves 3; best for the last two weeks of pregnancy

My baby is basking in my golden love.

Warming Cardamom Rose Milk

In Ayurveda, warm milks with ghee are prescribed to pacify any imbalances in vata and pitta doshas, which can cause unsettled sleep. They are a true comfort to the soul! Try sipping this heavenly combination of warm milk, ghee, cardamom, and rose petals in a pretty mug before bedtime and notice how your shoulders relax and the furrow in your brow softens. Choose the milk that works best for you—if you don't like or digest cow dairy well, any milk alternative will work here.

1 cup (240 ml) milk of choice (almond, cow, goat, macadamia, coconut, rice, oat)

1 teaspoon ghee

¼ teaspoon cardamom powder

1 tablespoon dry rose petals or 5 drops rose water

pinch of sea salt

OPTIONAL
honey

beet powder for a light pink color, if you have it

In a small pot over medium-high heat, bring milk to a quick boil, then turn off the heat and add ghee, cardamom, rose petals or rose water, and salt. Cover and steep for 20 minutes. Strain, add honey and beet powder (if using), and drink warm.

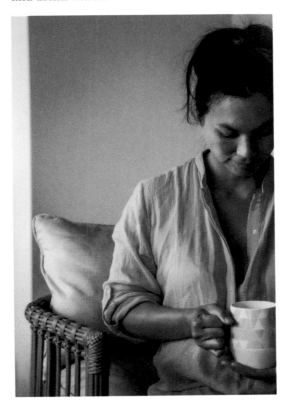

Serves 1; great in any trimester

My baby feels me and hears me.

Third Trimester Burdock Rose Tea

While in Maine at our photographer Jenny's house, I noticed she had a bag of burdock root in her pantry. The root had been grown and dried by a local herbalist and friend, Melissa Boynton of Natural Dawnings, and was calling to me to be steeped in tea. Mineral-rich burdock is known to balance blood sugar, stimulate digestion, and support the pancreas, and it is a gentle laxative too. We paired the root with delicate rose petals to create a tea that exemplified balance—burdock grounds you as your body morphs and changes, while the rose helps open the heart to embrace the new chapter to come. It's best to sip on this tea in late pregnancy as you prepare for the opening and release of birth.

3½ cups (840 ml) filtered water

1 tablespoon dry burdock root

1 tablespoon dry rose petals

Option 1: In a medium pot over medium-high heat, bring filtered water to a boil, add burdock and rose petals, turn off heat, and steep for 20 minutes with the lid on. Strain and sip throughout the day.

Option 2 (for deeper flavor): In a medium pot over medium-high heat, bring filtered water to a boil. Place burdock and rose petals into a 32-ounce (960 ml) glass Mason jar and pour in the hot water. Let it steep overnight and strain the next morning, then sip throughout the day.

Serves 2; best for third trimester

I am whole.

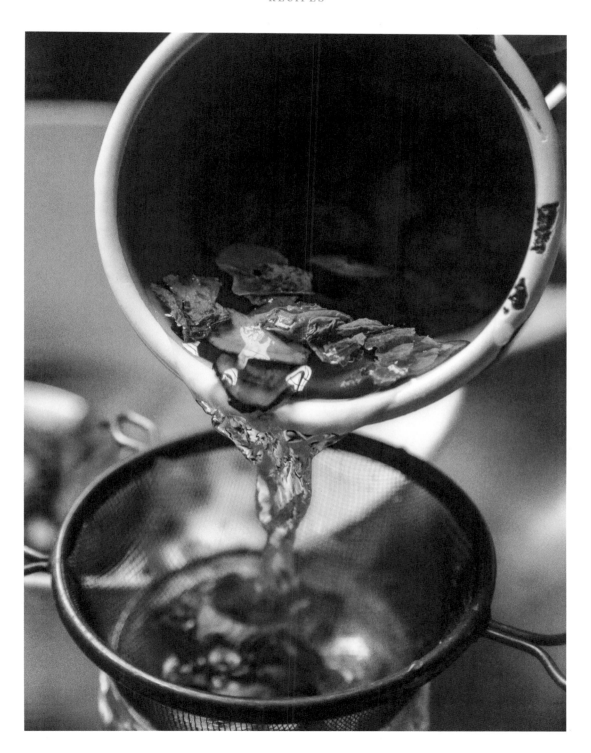

Stinging Nettle & Lemon Balm Tea

I have an enduring love affair with the nettle plant. Whether I find it dried at the natural grocers, on sale in fresh bunches in farmers' markets, or glimpse it in a friend's yard, growing wild as a weed, I'm always after it. (Wearing protective gloves if it's fresh, to avoid the prickly stingers!) I adore the flavor of it in tea, and I swear I can sense the infusion of vitamins and minerals into my cells as I drink it. The plant is a nutrient powerhouse, delivering vitamins A, B C, D and K, as well as calcium, iron, magnesium, and potassium in each sip. Nettle tea can help improve energy, strengthen blood vessels, reduce varicose veins, alleviate leg cramps, prevent anemia, and decrease the chances of hemorrhage after birth—so it's my most-recommended herb to use during pregnancy, and to continue using in the postpartum weeks as well! Here, it's blended with lemon balm, which helps soothe digestion and jagged nerves, and oat straw, which is rich in calcium and B vitamins and can help ease leg cramping and insomnia.

3½ cups (840 ml) filtered water

2 tablespoons dry stinging nettle leaves

2 tablespoons dry red raspberry leaves

2 tablespoons dry lemon balm

2 tablespoons dry oat straw

Option 1: In a medium pot over medium-high heat, bring filtered water to a boil, then add nettle and raspberry leaves, lemon balm, and oat straw, turn off heat, and steep for 20 minutes with the lid on. Strain and sip throughout the day.

Option 2 (for deeper flavor): In a medium pot over medium-high heat, bring filtered water to a boil. Place nettle and raspberry leaves, lemon balm, and oat straw into a 32-ounce (960 ml) glass Mason jar and pour in the hot water. Let it steep overnight and strain the next morning, then sip throughout the day.

All of these dried herbs and flowers are best sourced online. I recommend mountainroseherbs.com or oshalafarm.com.

Serves 2; best for second and third trimesters

My baby, you are my teacher. I am grateful for what you are teaching me.

Nourish You Tea

Starting in your second trimester, and throughout labor and postpartum, this tea is your ally. Red raspberry leaf is often called "the woman's herb" for its ability to support female reproductive health, soothe pregnancy discomforts, and help carry the baby to term. During pregnancy, it's particularly useful for uterine health and encouraging blood flow to the uterus, and it may reduce pain during labor and after birth. Mothers intending to do a VBAC (vaginal birth after cesarean) would do well to drink this tea! Enjoy 1 to 2 cups (240 to 480 ml) a day (you can refrigerate it in between servings). The tea leaves can be fed to your garden or houseplants after brewing. When you are closer to birth, say to yourself, "I am grateful this tea will nourish me and my baby and help support us with an easy birth."

3½ cups (840 ml) filtered water

1 tablespoon dry red raspberry leaves

1 tablespoon dry stinging nettle leaves

1 tablespoon dry oat straw

½ teaspoon local honey

Option 1: In a medium pot over medium-high heat, bring filtered water to a boil, then add raspberry and nettle leaves and oat straw, turn off heat, and steep for 20 minutes with the lid on. Strain, add honey, and sip throughout the day.

Option 2 (for deeper flavor): In a medium pot over medium-high heat, bring filtered water to a boil. Place raspberry and nettle leaves and oat straw into a 32-ounce (960 ml) glass Mason jar and pour in the hot water. Let steep overnight and strain the next morning, add honey, then sip throughout the day.

TEAS, TONICS & ELIXIRS

Serves 2; best for second and third trimesters

My ancestors surround me and support me.

Fresh Juice Recipes

I credit my love affair with healing foods to the first fresh juice I ever had, almost nineteen years ago while pregnant with my first child. I was gaining weight quickly in the first trimester, and my midwife, Davi, encouraged me to wean off the sweets I had grown accustomed to eating while living in England (pastries with my morning coffee, cookies later with my afternoon tea) and look for more healthful alternatives. This was easier than imagined, as I lived in the fresh juice mecca of the world—Los Angeles. I started with carrot and beet and worked my way up to kale, spinach, and the occasional shot of wheatgrass, visiting my local juicer almost daily. I welcomed the burst of flavor and the sense that my cells were receiving a direct dose of high-powered nutrition; soon, the buzz of the cold-press juicer became one of my favorite sounds (and the inspiration to buy my own home juicer). Most fruits, with the exception of low-glycemic berries, are extremely high in sugar (apples, beets, carrots), so whenever possible, stick with half an apple, leafy green veggies, and hydrating cucumbers. Juice shops can be found easily these days, but buying juice can be pricey, and there's nothing quite like being in command of your own experience. For at-home juicing, I suggest investing in a high quality juicer—it will save you money in the long run. My favorite? Omega Juicers' MM900HDS Low Speed Masticating. Remember to wash all fruits and vegetables well to avoid bacteria, including *E. coli*!

JUICE 1:
LEMON SPINACH
APPLE JUICE

1 large cucumber, peeled, quartered

½ red apple, peeled, sliced, de-seeded

½ lemon, peeled, quartered, de-seeded

1 cup (30 g) organic baby spinach

1 cup (45 g) organic baby kale

1 (¼-inch/6 mm) knob fresh ginger, halved

JUICE 2:
BEET CUCUMBER
MINT JUICE

1 medium red beet, peeled, quartered

½ red apple, peeled, de-seeded

1 large cucumber, peeled, quartered

½ cup (25 g) fresh mint

Juice each combination separately, alternating between the two each day. Ideally, drink shortly after juicing.

Serves 1

I open myself to birth when it is time.

Morning Sickness Elixir

Nausea during pregnancy is no fun. It can make you feel hypervigilant, wondering when the next wave will hit. In my own pregnancies, it was quite present. Looking back, I envision it shaking me up, waking me up to be fully present to the experience, but I still wanted to smooth out its rough edges whenever possible. Sipping on a drink full of electrolytes (charged minerals) can help maintain inner balance. This drink uses coconut water, celery, and cucumber juice, plus salt to hydrate and provide electrolytes, and ginger and lemon to further assist in calming the nausea. Feel free to leave out anything that doesn't appeal. Take small sips between waves of queasiness, doing your best to relax your shoulders and take deep breaths. Also try pressing on the acupressure point listed below, as acupuncture points are located throughout your body, connecting meridian lines to organs. This particular point is known to relieve nausea because the meridian pathway travels up the arm and into the chest and upper abdomen, near the stomach.

½ lemon, peeled, de-seeded

1 (¼-inch/6 mm) knob fresh ginger, peel on

1 celery stalk

1 large cucumber, peeled, quartered

½ apple, peeled, quartered

2 cups (480 ml) organic coconut water

pinch of sea salt

Juice lemon, ginger, celery, cucumber, apple.

Pour juice into a glass container and add coconut water and salt. Drink shortly after juicing.

Acupressure point: Open palm facing up. Measure with three fingers down from the top of your wrist. Press firmly for 2 to 3 minutes.

Serves 1

My body gratefully receives hydration.

Morning Sickness Warming Tea

Morning sickness affects 60 to 80 percent of pregnant women, and it can strike any time of the day or night, so it's good to have a couple of soothing options in your anti-nausea arsenal. When you're feeling green, choose between the Morning Sickness Elixir (page 241) and this soothing tea that marries ginger with chamomile, red raspberry, and a pop of fennel to calm your nerves and settle your belly. This tea is also a good option when drinking water feels like a chore, helping you get the fluids you need with a gentle hint of flavor.

3½ cups (840 ml) filtered water

1 tablespoon red raspberry leaves

1 tablespoon fennel seeds

1 tablespoon chamomile blossoms

1 (1-inch/2.5 cm) knob fresh ginger, skin on, sliced

1 teaspoon local honey

Option 1: In a medium pot over medium-high heat, bring filtered water to a boil, then add red raspberry leaves, fennel seeds, chamomile blossoms, and ginger. Turn off heat and steep for 20 minutes with the lid on. Strain, add honey, and sip throughout the day.

Option 2 (for deeper flavor): In a medium pot over medium-high heat, bring filtered water to a boil. Place red raspberry leaves, fennel seeds, chamomile blossoms, and ginger into a 32-ounce (960 ml) glass Mason jar and pour in the hot water. Let it steep overnight and strain the next morning, then sip at room temperature throughout the day.

Serves 2

I am powerful beyond my imagination.

Hydrating Berry Elixir

I remember a point right before the birth of my second baby when the light contractions I had come to count on—they meant our newest addition would be here soon!—suddenly stopped. Before I became alarmed, I remembered that hydration directly influences how we labor. I grabbed an electrolyte beverage and after a few big sips, my contractions returned. The uterus, like many muscles, functions most properly when it is fully hydrated, and electrolytes help the body maintain a proper fluid level. Luckily, you don't have to guzzle a big-name sports drink with artificial sugar and color to receive the benefits of electrolytes. This version offers all the goodness of a store-bought beverage—namely, some calories and deep hydration—with no unwelcome additives, plus a touch of strawberry to sweeten your experience. Lemon adds vitamin C, and the electrolytes come from a hearty sprinkling of ConcenTrace® Trace Mineral Drops. (You can find them at natural food markets or online.) I've been told that sipping on this elixir throughout active labor can give you a boost of stamina when you may need it most.

2 quarts (2 L) filtered water

1 (1½-inch/4 cm) knob fresh ginger, grated

½ to 1 cup (120 to 240 ml) honey (depends on how sweet you like it)

juice of 1 lemon

2 cups (250 g) strawberries, sliced

6 drops to 1 teaspoon ConcenTrace® Trace Mineral Drops or pinch of sea salt

In a medium pot over medium-high heat, bring water to a boil. Add grated ginger, turn off the heat, and let it brew for 20 minutes, then strain. Stir in honey.

Wait for the tea to cool down, then add lemon juice, strawberry slices, and trace mineral drops or salt and stir.

Allow the strawberries to infuse for 1 hour, then strain to avoid bits in your drink.

Store in a glass Mason jar in the refrigerator or in the freezer.

Freezing tip: Fill one 16- or 32-ounce (480 or 960 ml) glass Mason jar, leaving 1 inch (2.5 cm) of room at the top for expansion, and place in the freezer without lids. Once frozen, place the lids on. This will prevent glass from cracking. Freeze for up to 2 months.

Note: During labor, I highly recommend using a bendy straw. It will make it much easier to sip between contractions.

TEAS, TONICS & ELIXIRS

Makes 8 cups (2 L)

I am quietly listening to you, baby.

SNACKS

Try these quick homemade snacks instead of a packaged or processed choice.

- Spread tahini on apple slices and add a drizzle of honey.

- Cut a celery stalk into segments and spread with almond butter.

- Peel one "side" of a banana, smother with almond butter, remove remaining peel, and cut banana into slices.

- Smother a baked yam with pasture-raised or vegan butter (I recommend Miyoko's Creamery) and sprinkle with ume plum vinegar.

- Slice a delicata squash, seeds intact, into ¼-inch (6 mm) circles, drizzle with oil, season with salt, then roast for 30 to 40 minutes, until slightly crisp and caramelized.

- Slice 2 Persian cucumbers and top with a mixture of 1 teaspoon sesame oil, 1 tablespoon coconut aminos, ¼ teaspoon ume plum vinegar, and white sesame seeds.

- Top 2 cups (120 g) summer sugar snap peas with 1 teaspoon lemon juice and a pinch of sea salt. Cover and steam for 2 minutes.

- Spread butter on rice crackers, followed by chicken liver pâté, pickled herring, and cucumber pickles.

- Mix organic popcorn with 3 tablespoons pasture-raised or vegan butter (such as Miyoko's Creamery), 4 to 6 tablespoons (55 to 85 g) nutritional yeast, 1 tablespoon Hawaiian spirulina powder, and sea salt. (Note: Pop your own kernels in a heavy-bottomed pan, covered, over medium-high heat, using a generous tablespoon of coconut oil or butter.)

- Stuff mini sweet bell peppers with a mixture of cashew cheese or cottage cheese, everything bagel seasoning, and lemon juice.

- Top half an avocado with extra-virgin olive oil, black pepper, lemon juice, and a hard-boiled egg, sprinkled with sea salt.

- Spoon Wild Blueberry Compote (see page 215) over a small bowl of cottage cheese.

- Have some jerky: beef, buffalo, elk, wild boar, or salmon.

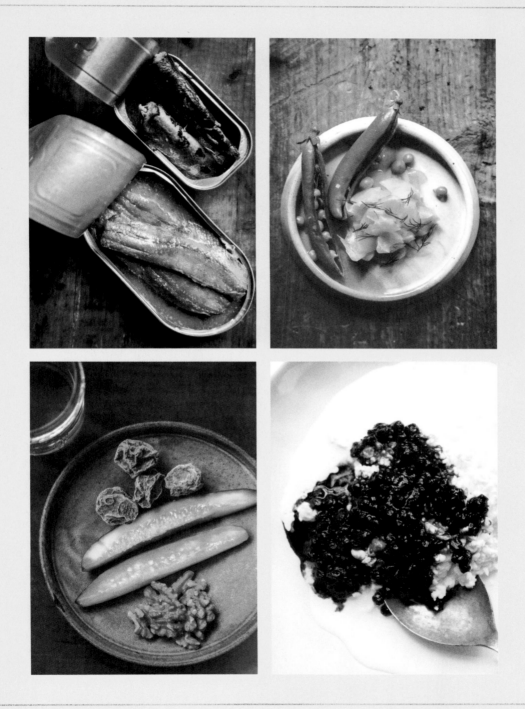

BODY CARE

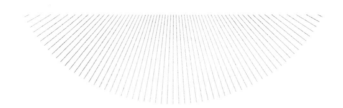

Ginger Foot Bath

In Chinese medicine, the body is often compared to a tree. The torso represents the trunk, and the hands and feet are the roots, making them a critical site of health and vitality. This simple foot bath is a clear act of honoring the part of your body that has been dutifully carrying you and your baby. In taking the time to soak your feet, you are dropping into a beautiful place of non-doing for at least a few moments and claiming some much-needed time for *you*. Soaking your feet before bed can also help support a good night's rest. As a gesture of love and respect, your partner or a good friend can pour this foot bath for you before you climb into bed.

6 (2-inch/5 cm) knobs fresh ginger, skin on, sliced

In a medium pot over medium-high heat, bring 3 quarts (2.8 L) water to a boil and add ginger. Reduce the heat to medium-low and simmer for an additional 30 minutes. Turn off heat and leave to cool until lukewarm.

Strain ginger water into a foot bath or a large bowl and soak your feet for 20 minutes. Add additional hot water as needed.

Note: This is only to be used as a foot bath; it is not a tea to be consumed.

BODY CARE

My thoughts and emotions are mine to process and not my baby's to carry.

Baths for a Queen

When you put your phone on silent, pop a "Do not disturb" sign on the bathroom door, and draw a warm bath, you are choosing yourself in a bold way. I like to bump up my bath experience with sea salts, dry herbs, candles, meditation music, and fresh rose petals if possible—simple ways to feel like a queen. These two baths are a direct route to stress relief. The recipes can be made in advance, stored in jars, and refrigerated until you're ready to decompress. (Preparing in advance means no pesky herbs to pull out of the drain post bath.) For both, fill the tub with warm—not scalding hot—water, add the herbal soak or milk and honey mixture, then gently lower yourself into the bath. Give yourself a moment to adjust to the warmth, then close your eyes and feel your worries and responsibilities gently fade away. When you are finished, drain the tub and thank the water for washing away the stress of the day. As it gets more difficult to bend over in the third trimester, practice asking a loved one to draw a bath for you.

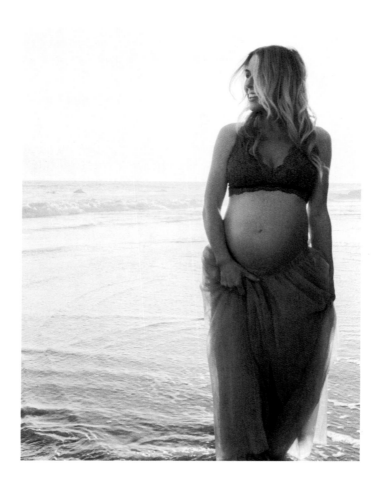

ROSE HONEY MILK BATH

For centuries, milk and honey have been a revered beauty combo known for soothing and softening the skin. It's easy to see why—the lactic acid in milk gently removes dead skin cells, and honey is a natural humectant, keeping skin moist but not oily. To make this bath the ultimate in skin soothing experiences, I added oatmeal, which calms dry, irritated skin. Finally, I sprinkled in my all-time favorite—rose petals (I just can't get enough!)—to open the heart and cultivate a sense of self-love.

2 cups (180 g) rolled oats

2 cups (65 g) dry rose petals (I order these from Mountain Rose Herbs at mountainroseherbs.com)

4 cups (960 ml) cow milk

1 cup (240 ml) honey

24 fresh rose petals (optional)

In a large pot over medium-high heat, add oats, dry rose petals, milk, and 4 cups (960 ml) water and bring to a light boil. Reduce the heat to medium-low and simmer for 30 minutes, until the oats cook down and the mixture takes on a milky rose tea color.

Strain the mixture into a large pitcher, stir in the honey, and pour contents into your warm bath water (or pour into jars and store in the fridge for later). To make it extra delightful, add a handful of fresh rose petals to the tub.

Makes 1 bath

My baby glows with pure love.

HERBAL SOAK

This combination of warm water and fresh flowers and herbs is downright magical. Lavender is deeply relaxing, and chamomile soothes sensitive skin. I suggest soaking for 20 to 30 minutes to bring renewed energy and clarity, soothe nerves, and soften muscles—just what your hard-working pregnant body is crying out for. For an extra pop of beauty, sprinkle in a few rose petals right before sliding into the tub. If it is winter, use dried flowers or herbs.

6 cups (1.4 L) boiling water

1 cup (30 g) fresh or dry lavender

1 cup (30 g) fresh or dry chamomile flowers

2 cups (65 g) dry rose petals or 1 cup (95 g) ground rose petals (I order these from Mountain Rose Herbs at mountainroseherbs.com.)

Fill two 32-ounce (960 ml) wide-mouthed glass jars or a medium pot with the boiling water. With your hands, gently crush the flowers and herbs into the water, stirring with a spoon and holding an intention for what you would like to receive from the bath. Less pain in your body? Happy relationships with your family? An easeful birth? Or you may simply wish for your mind and muscles to deeply unwind. Let the flowers and herbs steep in water for 3 hours.

Strain, compost the remains, and store the flower and herbal water in jars in the fridge until you are ready to use. Pour both jars into a warm bath when you are ready to lovingly tend to yourself.

Makes 1 soak

Love flows from and through me.

Massage Oil: Breast Care

I never considered breast massage until a massage therapist asked me if she could work on that part of my body during a session. I understood that this was one of her areas of expertise, so I set aside any awkwardness and said yes. Breast tissue is usually not touched unless you are breastfeeding or in an intimate encounter, and I was surprised to find the experience extremely invigorating. Turns out, breast massage is a wonderful way to stimulate the nerves, lymph nodes, and tissues, and to release stagnant energy. Massaging the breasts is also a wonderful way to give yourself the gift of self-love, honoring this powerful part of your body with some dedicated TLC—before its primary purpose becomes feeding your baby.

The breasts contain a variety of glands that benefit from stimulation—as my midwife, Davi, says, what better time to "get to know your girlfriends" than now? Proceed gently, as your breast tissue may be sore from engorgement; even slight pressure and movements can bring some relief.

Start with a carrier oil from the list below and add a few drops of the essential oil of your choice.

1 tablespoon carrier oil of choice (almond, coconut, sesame)

3 to 4 drops essential oil of choice (calendula, grapefruit, lavender, rose)

In a small bowl, combine carrier oil and essential oil and stir well.

Find a comfortable, quiet space and set an intention.

With your fingers, scoop oil onto one breast and move in a circular motion from the outside, in, toward your nipple. Make sure to engage the armpit, where many glands and breast tissue are located, taking slow, deep breaths.

Gently move onto your other breast and repeat.

After the second breast is massaged, place one hand on the outside of each breast, move them inward and across, toward each other like a figure eight. Repeat several times, breathing with your eyes closed.

Makes 1 potion; best during the last two weeks of pregnancy, to put support and intention behind milk coming in for baby

I love all of you. I love all of me.

Acknowledgments

THIS BOOK IS DEDICATED TO TU-QUYEN DAM, my maternal grandmother, affectionately known as Po-Po. With her mother's support, Po-Po had aspired to study medicine after high school, but due to the invasion of Japan in China, the journey from Hong Kong to Beijing was too unsafe for a young, single woman. Her wishes faded to an unattainable dream while her eldest brother continued on to study law. The whispers of her wisdom and sacrifice have motivated and informed the creation of each of my books, along with those of her Chinese-born grandfather-in-law and mentor Dr. Huang (1869–1952), who famously healed his community in Vietnam with his herbal formulations.

I am also eternally grateful to my children, Khefri, India, and Jude—who are my life-long teachers—as well as my midwife, Davi Khalsa, and doula, Khefri Riley, who have taught me so much about pregnancy, birth, and motherhood and continue to inspire me today.

*Nine Golden Month*s would not exist without my treasured co-authors, Amely Greeven and Marisa Belger, who poured their hearts and souls into its creation, even while the world was more unsettled than ever. They bring so much valuable experience from their own mothering journeys and such gifts of writerly wisdom to each of our books. Our collaboration is precious and gets richer with each project we embark on together.

I offer deep gratitude to the wise ones who generously contributed their expansive knowledge to this book. It is an honor to be able to share your insights with so many readers across the globe.

To my photographers, Jenny McNulty of Wylde Photography, Stephanie Entin of Little Plum Photography, and Khefri Wilcox—your work played a key role in creating an exquisite atmosphere for our readers. It was a joy to work side by side, creating each shot together, and I thank you for your patience with my perfectionism. Cheers, also, to Jessica Janney, whose invaluable guidance helped shape the recipe section; and Dana LaRue Park, for your eagle-eyed editing. Thank you, Michelle Blandina, Leah and Rod Arzu, and Belinda Gosbee, for your beautiful belly shots.

This book is the third baby in a family that was conceived from a very personal idea—creating a guide for new mothers finding their way during the unpredictable early days after giving birth. I'm in awe of what that small idea has grown into! Thank you to my editor Holly Dolce and the entire ABRAMS team, and my editor Marc Gerald and his wife, Christina. You all believed in this vision from the very beginning, and your belief in me gave me all the more confidence in myself.

Last but certainly not least, thank you to my MotherBees community and all the birth workers who inspire me every day. Your support helps me give voice to the stories and wisdom of my lineage. I believe my ancestors would be extremely proud.

Recipe Index

Index

Editor: Holly Dolce
Designer: Laura Palese
Design Manager: Danielle Youngsmith
Managing Editor: Annalea Manalili
Production Manager: Kathleen Gaffney

Library of Congress Control Number: 2022932169

ISBN: 978-1-4197-5148-6
eISBN: 978-1-64700-185-8

ABRAMS The Art of Books
195 Broadway, New York, NY 10007
abramsbooks.com